Table of Contents

Introduction

The science of gerontology has been jokingly referred to as of interest primarily to biologists approaching retirement. This was not true in my case. In 1941 I published an article in my high school magazine, *The Literary Parade*, in which I deplored the brevity of life. To me, even a fairly long life seemed far too short to explore the world's outward wonders and humankind's inner realms, to walk all the strange pathways of society's subcultures, to read all the books, hear all the music, climb the mountains and dive the seas, to be present at least at the early stages of the age of space.

Does this sound sophomoric? Maybe so. But I still feel that way. "Life piled on life were all too little," to quote "Ulysses," a poem by Tennyson. And curiously enough, as my daughter and I finished writing this book, fifty-three years after the dreams and fantasies of high school days, I was engaged at all levels in a sort of "Anti-Aging Odyssey." Sealed inside Biosphere 2 in the Arizona desert along with seven others, I saw how "Life piled on life" makes living a greatly extended healthy life an attractive option.

I confess that at first gerontology seemed just a means to an end. I simply wanted to live longer, to have it all and do it all. As an honors student entering the California Institute of Technology (CalTech), I was more into mathematics and philosophy. But Descartes, who was preeminent in both of these fields, died at fifty-two. That would be awful, I figured. And so I set out *not* to die at fifty-two, or even twice that. And I was determined to have a great, productive, zestful time of it, for *all* of that time.

But a deep interest in biology began to push itself forward, until ... but here I must tell you a story.

I was a 19-year-old student at CalTech. One weekend I was at a field station laboratory. We were taking a tea break on the first-floor balcony, which the wild woodland marched right up to. And here he was: Nobel Laureate Sir Thomas Hunt Morgan, the great founder of the genetic edifice of the fruit fly (*Drosophila melanogaster*). As I stood there, wide-eyed, regarding him with deep respect, this illustrious old man leaned over the balcony railing, intensely watching a salamander on a twig. The salamander was laying eggs one by one into a gel matrix, which she was also secreting, to form a translucent amber egg sac stuck fast to the twig.

Now, salamanders and egg-laying had nothing to do with why Sir Thomas was there that afternoon, but after a time I saw him straighten up, and I heard him mutter to himself as though he had waited all his life for that moment, "Ah ha! So that's how she does it!"

And that's how life does it, life piled on life or simply sitting on a twig.

Old Sir Thomas had impressed me deeply. It was one of those moments when you seem to step through a curtain and a transformation starts that — on the surface — has nothing to do with you, but of which you are the center. And then Sir Thomas winked. One eye remained fixed on the salamander, the other eye twitched and seemed to wink marvelously at me. His enthusiasm, for the secrets of life's complex processes, had become mine. It was a great gift, and I like to think that it was done on purpose by a kind, great mind.

So biology came alive for me — for more than simply exploiting it to extend my own life and stay vigorous and healthy.

I graduated from medical school at the University of Chicago in 1948 and headed, along with my lifelong friend, NASA's Dr. Albert Hibbs, for . . . the gambling casinos of Nevada. Remember my conviction that long life, to be well lived, must be punctuated with adventure, with varieties of experience. (I was captain of the wrestling team at the University of Chicago for two years, missing Olympic tryouts because of an injured shoulder — and always regretted missing the Olympic experience, since I had come reasonably close.) Al and I wanted to sail the Caribbean before going on with our scientific careers. To buy a sailboat we needed money. In Reno and Las Vegas we parlayed a roulette system we devised into fairly big bucks. This brought us a surprising amount of publicity — a full page in *Life Magazine* and all that, and when I did receive my M.D. degree, the Chicago paper carried the caption "Gambling Ace Wins M.D."

So we bought our boat and sailed the Caribbean, but that's another story. There followed an internship at the famous Gorgas Hospital in Panama, then residency training, then two years as an Air Force physician during the Korean War. In 1954 I joined the faculty at UCLA School of Medicine. It was time to get serious about gerontology as a biologic discipline, about health enhancement, about extending the vitality of youth and middle age to over the hundred-year mark.

In the course of my long stay at UCLA — during which, by means of a good wife (now divorced) and some confused help from me, three fine children were raised — I've spent year-long periods (sabbatical years) elsewhere, often as a sort of scientist-adventurer. A year in Freiburg, Germany, by the Black Forest, which in 1960 was still pristine and beautiful, not blasted by industrial pollution as it is now. Paris in 1968, at the laboratory of Nobelist Jean Dausset, during which time I covered the student revolution for the *Los Angeles Free Press*, and associated intimately with and wrote about the Living Theater (they have been a major influence in my life: another story). A year wandering around India looking for ancient wisdom, or even modern wisdom — and finding some of both. In 1983, trekking and hitchhiking across central Africa. And finally the grand living experiment of Biosphere 2, which combined science and adventure as never before.

But mainly, time was spent at UCLA, focused upon my developing research laboratory. During my watch, gerontology has moved from the fringes of science to its present position, center stage with its own institute at the National Institutes of Health. With its promise of a major extension in human life span, an event so far-reaching in its effect on society that it will rank with mankind's change from a hunter-gatherer to an agricultural, industrial, and now an information-based society. Many of those now alive will be participating in this vast change.

My work in gerontology at UCLA took a number of exciting directions: how the immune system varies in aging and perhaps is partly responsible for aging; the genetics of aging, i.e., what genes regulate aging; how cells age in tissue culture, i.e., "under glass" in the laboratory; and finally, what has proven the most immediately applicable to human aging: the caloric limitation experiments that form the subject of this book.

All the early work had been done in animals. In Biosphere 2, I had begun one of my adventure-scientist's side trips: to be the physician inside for a two-year sealed-in cruise. But what I had walked into innocently turned out to be a one-in-a-million happy trick of fate. Here in Biosphere 2 I had the opportunity to test the effect of a high-quality but calorically limited diet in humans, and under closely monitored conditions — to gain evidence that the results I had already obtained in animals would be applicable to humans.

Biosphere 2 is a massive closed ecological space on the Arizona desert near Tucson. It houses over 3,800 carefully selected species of plants and animals and is watched over by a crew (also carefully selected!) of specialists I'll call Biospherians. No exchanges with the outside world were to be permitted. Biosphere 2 was to be electronically open, but closed to exchange of any physical material, including even atmospheric gases, with the outside world. If you were as small as an electron, you could come and go at will, as big as a molecule, no luck. (This policy held for the first year, but was then modified to permit exchange of scientific specimens through an airlock.) Inside Biosphere 2 we had to grow all our own food, recycle all wastes. That was the arrangement.

We found that we could only grow food enough to provide each Biospherian with about 1,800 calories per day for the first six months. But the diet was high in overall quality.

To the extent that I was able to measure, I found the same changes in the Biospherians on a calorically limited diet as I had previously found in animals: changes in blood pressure, cholesterol, blood sugar, and the number of white cells in the blood, and in general health, disease resistance, and vitality. These parallel changes strongly supported the inference that the other effects — the across-the-board health enhancement and the aging retardation — would also occur. My results on the Biospherians, myself included, were published in the December 1992 issue of the *Proceedings of the National Academy of Sciences*.

The diet and background for the present book come from the overall, long-term experiments I've mentioned above, in Biospherians and in animals. Recent and ongoing studies in monkey colonies point in the same direction. Ordinarily, a high-quality (we use the term "nutrient rich"), low-calorie diet can require a lot of cooking — can be labor intensive, so to speak. And that's just not practical in today's busy world. In this book my daughter, Lisa Walford, and I have therefore shouldered the task of making the diet simple and doable, as well as tasty. You'll like it. You'll lose weight and you'll feel healthier, more energized. Your resistance to diseases like the common cold will increase. Your skin, if you have acne, will clear up, as it did in two Biospherians. And other health benefits will accrue, as we will show. Become your own adventure-scientist, and with our confident blessing.

--RLW, *UCLA Medical School*

We are grateful to the following people who helped us in the creation of this book: Ian Berger, Cynthia Cameros, Frances Jalet-Miller, Brian Lee, Elinor Nauen, Naomi Rosenblatt, Dan Simon, Lynn Theard, John Thomas, Margery Tippie, Martha Walford, and Larry Weber.

--RLW and LW, *Venice, CA*

BOOK ONE

STRATEGIES

Chapter 1

The Biosphere Experience

The actual diet eaten by the Biospherians during the two years sealed inside was high in quality (we can refer to this as nutrient rich, which means each calorie is packed with nutrition) and low in calories, but quite limited in variety. It's not very satisfying to have sweet potatoes as part of every meal — breakfast, lunch, and dinner — for two to three straight months, just because they are growing well during that season. (We became very ingenious at preparing sweet potatoes in different ways — as custards mixed with bananas, as roasted slices, baked whole, and so on). Another of our seasons might be extra heavy on beets — even harder to prepare in different ways.

All Biospherians cooked. Every eighth day you had to prepare breakfast, lunch, and dinner for the whole crew. Almost every breakfast included a porridge made from whole-wheat flour and bananas. The wheat had to be grown, harvested, threshed, and ground, all by us. And that's just a small task when you're running a whole mini-world.

Table 1.1 shows what and how much was eaten by each Biospherian on eight representative days. Crops in Biosphere 2 were planned so that a complete nutritional complement was always available (the nutrient-rich calorie), despite changing crop cycles. There were six varieties of fruit (banana, fig, guava, lemon, papaya, kumquat), five cereal grains (oats, rice, sorghum, wheat, corn), split

Table 1.1: REPRESENTATIVE DAILY INTAKES OVER TWO YEARS IN BIOSPHERE 2 ((GIVEN AS TWO RANDOM DAYS FROM EACH OF THE FOUR SIX MONTH PERIODS)) *

FOODS	AMOUNT (IN GRAMS)							
banana	375	197	281	260	254	225	263	319
fig		66	40					
guava		13		8	5			
lemon	12		6	10	5	12	10	
papaya			169	152	35	131		186
kumquat		16						
peanuts	25	18	15	18	18	18	18	68
rice	57	102			57	57		57
sorghum	40			70	70			
wheat	75	76	198	73	73	153	153	96
corn,		17						
beans,								
dried	36							
lablab	36	28	28					57
pinto	9			50			57	
soy	9				29	57		
string				26	15	37		
peas, split	18							
beets	225	281				153	90	118
beet greens						84	40	
bok choi			90					
cabbage	125					108		
carrots	48	86	20				150	
chard	188	86		125	33	46	67	
eggplant	56				14	37	60	80
cucumber						63	60	
herbs	2	15						
lettuce	63	46	8	64	40		37	23
malanga		143	280					115
onions		99	66	10	17	18	12	
parsley				5	2		4	
pepper, green		4		84	73	82	24	50
pepper, red	2							20
potato, swt	300			519	468	552	630	411
potato, wht		236	239					
raddish					48			
squash		241	394	238	42	71	78	25
tomato	58	321	30	60		84	28	
turnip grns		60						
eggs				30				
goat milk	100	50	70	150	100	165	235	150
pork			43					
total cal	1825	1863	1910	2201	1935	2190	2140	2274
fat, gms	27	19	22	39	36	37	30	51
protein	62	60	68	69	56	78	70	73
carb	370	360	395	434	327	432	440	425
fiber, gms	48	61	55	52	44	61	55	48

* Additional foods available at various times, but not used on these 8 random days, included oats, millet, kidney beans, lima beans, kale fresh peas, sweet potatoe greens, purslane, turnips, raddishes, chicken, fish (talapia), goat meat, and yogurt.

peas, peanuts, five varieties of beans, nineteen vegetables and greens, white and sweet potatoes, *small* quantities of goat milk and yogurt, and one weekly serving of 3.5-ounce quantities of goat meat, pork, chicken, or fish, and one egg-per-week. As you can see, the variety was limited, and the calorie content low — especially in relation to the great physical labor involved in running Biosphere 2 — but the "quality" of the diet was nutrient rich, judging by computer analyses of the content of vitamins, minerals, and other essential nutrients. And the diet induced remarkable and beneficial changes in the Biospherians, which we shall be detailing in this book. But it wasn't much fun, eating the same food combinations for two years, period. So the anti-aging diet we present here is not the Biospherian diet. The scientific principles are the same, and both derive ultimately from animal nutrition studies going back over half a century. The Anti-Aging Plan is a gourmet version, an easier-to-cook expression of this accumulated knowledge. It is low in calories and fat, high in nutrient quality (the nutrient-rich calorie), satisfying, tasty, and easy to prepare.

Five days after leaving the Biosphere, (called reentry by the lay press), I returned to conduct a group of physicians on a tour. I remember being amazed, incredulous even, that the eight of us — such a small number indeed — had actually been able to run this complex mini-world with all its gadgets, pipes, wiring, computer systems, to say nothing of the plants and animals . . . for two whole years. We were the crack shakedown crew, and in due course some intriguing psychological papers will emerge from the experience.

Chapter 2

Extending Your Healthy Years

The three top killers of adults are heart disease, stroke, and cancer, followed by the combination of pneumonia, influenza, and bronchitis, then accidents, diabetes, arteriosclerosis, and liver disease. We can predict with a margin of error of only 5 percent that you'll die of one of these diseases.

On the Anti-Aging Plan with caloric limitation, many fewer persons will be afflicted by these diseases, and if a disease does come, it will come later in life, at a time corresponding to *functional* age rather than *chronological* or *birthday* age. If a disease you might be due to get at age 50 doesn't appear until age 60, that's a ten-year cure, simply by preventive nutrition. And some nonkilling but troublesome maladies, like osteoporosis and arthritis, will very likely also be delayed by the Anti-Aging Plan.

Let's discuss some of these diseases, starting with the top killer of all:

Heart Disease and Arteriosclerosis

Percentages of all deaths from heart disease by age group are given in Figure 2.1. Deaths at younger ages are mainly comprised of congenital heart disease, rheumatic heart disease, and such, but beyond age forty-five arteriosclerosis of the heart's blood vessels is almost always the underlying cause. Studies in rodents, primates (monkeys), and humans, including most recently the Biospherians, all agree that this top killer is mostly caused by improper diet, and can be prevented or even reversed, by the Anti-Aging Plan. Elevated blood cholesterol is a major factor in causing artereosclerosis. Average values in Americans are much too high in all age groups and both sexes. However, those in the lowest 5 percent range tend to be free of heart disease. Certain isolated native populations also show very low blood cholesterol levels and very little artereosclerotic heart disease. The Tarahumara Indians of Mexico have a very low fat diet and adult cholesterol levels of 137; the Yanamomes of Brazil on a similiar diet show average levels of 133.

The Biospherian blood cholesterols before entry were 191. Six months later the average value was 123. No other dietary or drug regime has ever been shown to exert a comparable effect in Western industrialized societies.

High Blood Pressure

A stroke comes either from stoppage of blood flow to part of the brain — a clogging of the arteries secondary to arteriosclerosis — or a rupture of blood vessels due to high blood pressure, or a combination of these.

When your doctor measures your blood pressure, he records it as two numbers, for example 140/90. The upper number, called the systolic pressure, is the pressure the blood exerts on the arterial walls during the heartbeat. The lower, or distolic pressure, is the pressure remaining in the arteries between heartbeats. In adults, a pressure exceeding 140 systolic and/or 90 diastolic is the lowest rung of the hypertension ladder.

Among the Biospherians the average preentry value was 110/75, an overall normal value. On the Biospherian version of the Anti-Aging Plan, nevertheless, average blood pressure decreased steadily and by three months was 90/58. The blood pressure of the Biospherian who entered with a value of 130/90 (borderline diastolic hypertension) declined to 110/70. The blood pressures remained at these healthy lower values over the whole two years of the stay inside Biosphere 2.

Cancer

Here the evidence for the benefits of a high-quality, nutrient-rich, calorie-limited diet is overwhelming, both as to total incidence of cancers of most types, and time of occurrence in life (much later in animals on the nutrient-rich, calorie-limited diet!). Unfortunately we have no Biospherian data, as two years is too short a time for a cancer study. But animal evidence is almost certainly applicable to the human situation.

Table 2.1 summarizes information from studies in different university laboratories. All these studies concerned spontaneous cancers, i.e., those not related to the experimental application of some cancer-causing agent. The studies were done in mice of different inbred strains selected to have high incidence of the different cancers.

The beneficial effect of nutrient-dense caloric restriction on different kinds of cancer does vary. Cancer of the breast seems very significantly inhibited by nutrient-rich calorie restriction, cancer of the liver less so.

Table 2.1. INCIDENCE OF VARIOUS SPONTANEOUS CANCERS IN MICE ON AN ANTI-AGING DIET COMPARED TO AD LIB FED MICE. RESULTS FROM FOUR DIFFERENT STUDIES ARE PRESENTED.

Study	Type of Cancer	% in Ad Lib Fed	% in Restricted
#1	Breast	40	2
	Lung	60	30
#2	Breast	67	0
#3	Leukemia	65	10
#4	Liver	64	11

In spontaneous cancers, it is difficult to determine the time of onset, but you can determine the age(s) at which animals die from each type of cancer. In one study at the UCLA School of Medicine among mice ultimately dying from lymphatic cancer, those on a nutrient-rich, low-calorie diet survived eight to twelve months longer. This suggests that their tumors began at a much later birthday age. Eight to twelve months is one third the normal life span of a mouse, and would correspond to a fifteen-to-thirty-year postponement of cancer onset in humans. Among mice dying of liver cancer, those on the nutrient-rich, calorie-limited diet were six to fifteen months older at the time of death than regularly fed mice with similar cancers.

Other Age Related Diseases

Animals on a nutrient-rich, low-calorie diet do not show the bone loss usually seen in late life. These results suggest that persons on a nutrient-rich but calorically limited diet might be less susceptible to osteoporosis later in life.

Half of all Americans over fifty years of age have diverticulae (balloonlike outpouchings caused by excess pressure) in their large bowels, and a fraction of these persons develop the bloating, gas, nausea, cramping, and constipation that characterize diverticulitis. The Anti-Aging Plan, rich in both soluble and insoluble fibers, will help prevent diverticulitis.

Looks

Here again it is hard to draw convincing conclusions on the basis of a two-year experiment. Two Biospherians had severe acne on entering Biosphere 2. This cleared rapidly on the Biosphere diet. Others looked trimmer and more vital as they gradually lost weight, kept it off, and their body fat redistributed itself. In long-term animal experiments, a clearer picture emerges. Thirty-six months is extreme old age for fully fed mice. Their fur is in poor condition, heavily streaked with gray, they cease grooming themselves and develop hunched arthritic backs, and seem "shriveled up" as they approach great functional age, just like people. But calorie-limited mice of the same chronological age look (and test) young and agile.

Brain Function

Probably the greatest fear about growing old is the possibility of serious mental decline: forgetting things, being confused in public, and much worse. The extent to which this really happens, and especially the time of onset of the decline, is a subject of debate. Whatever the details may be, however, and judging again by animal data, the decline can be slowed, even largely prevented, by the Anti-Aging Plan with caloric limitation.

Mental function in laboratory animals can be estimated by their ability to navigate a complicated maze or labyrinth. How many trials does it take to learn when to choose this turn, that turn, and not end in blind alleys; and finally to arrive at the reward at the end of the maze? On such a test, a 32-month-old calorie-restricted mouse does as well as a 12-month-old ad lib mouse. This is roughly equivalent to a 75-year-old human showing the same speed of learning and same memory retention as a 25-year-old. And in rats the age-related slowdown in rate of learning and in memory utilization are largely eliminated by nutrient-rich caloric limitation.

Sexuality

Sexual activity can be taken as a rough measure of functional age, but the time of reproductive senescence is a more definite measure: We call it menopause in human females, and age-related infertility in mice. In mice, nutrient-rich, calorie-limited animals are still sexually active long after control (regularly fed) animals have ceased being so. Indeed, in some studies calorie-limited animals are still capable of bearing offspring when *all* the regularly fed animals have grown old and died. In one remarkable study, when regularly fed female animals already *past* the reproductive age were placed on high-quality calorie limitation for ten weeks, and then allowed full access to food for a brief period, they recommenced sexual activity and became pregnant. So maybe you can't take it with you, but you can keep it with you longer. Indeed, it is quite possible that a period of controlled high-quality calorie limitation followed by splurging might be of use in certain kinds of human infertility. Probably the limitation/refeeding technique stimulates ovulation.

The Internal Machinery of the Body

The immune system's response to challenges by bacterial or viral infections, the liver's ability to detoxify poisons, the kidney's blood-clearing functions, the integrity of the connective tissue, the hormonal systems of the body, the processes by which your body repairs its own DNA (the famous double helix that contains the genetic code) — these are all influenced in a highly favorable way by the Anti-Aging Plan, and extensive studies have confirmed that the immune system, whose functional capacity declines very substantially with normal aging, is kept "younger" longer by nutrient-rich calorie limitation.

Life Span

Your potential average and maximum life spans will be substantially increased by the nutrient-rich Anti-Aging Plan.

Let's say that your hereditary potential — the age you might expect to reach based upon the genes you've inherited from your parents — is to live to be 80 years old. Let's assume that you started and stuck to a rather high percentage of caloric limitation, beginning at age 20. Over that remaining 60 years you might expect to age at half the expected rate, be "functionally" 50 when you were in fact chronologically 80. Your 60 years would thus stretch out to 120. Add that to your initial 20 years (when you started) and you reach 140. And note that when you were in fact 100 years of age, you would "functionally" and in all outward appearances and inward workings be only 60.

Of course, even if this analysis holds in a population, one cannot guarantee that you as an individual will live to be 140. You will simply have skipped onto the survival curve of a population whose last surviving members live that long. Exactly when you personally might fall off that greatly extended curve can't be foretold. But you will be substantially younger in form, feature, and function than your birthday age. The evidence makes this relatively certain.

Naturally, if you choose a lower percentage of caloric limitation of the Anti-Aging Plan you won't obtain quite such amazing results, but you'll still be way ahead, even with no more than a 10 to 20 percent cutback. Pick the tradeoff that leaves you comfortable. We recommend that you try about a 20 percent restriction, and see how it goes. More is too much, unless you are under very close medical supervision.

Danger Signals and Don'ts

Do not lose more than 20 to 25 percent of your initial body weight, as an upper limit. Of course if you are slender to start with, even that would be too much. You have to use judgment, and consult with your doctor. The Biospherian men lost an average of 18 percent body weight, the women 10 percent. This was enough to induce in all of them psysiological changes that suggest retarded aging. Body fat content of the men declined to 6 to 10 percent; of women to10 to 15 percent. These should be taken as lower limits.

If you are a woman and weight loss becomes associated with any menstrual irregularities, that's too fast or too much. Consult your doctor. None of the Biospherian women experienced menstrual irregularities.

If you find yourself having to sleep longer than usual, or becoming fatigued or light-headed, you have lost weight too fast or too much. Proper use of the diet should do the reverse of these things. Be sure your diet is high in quality, not just low in calories!

Functional Age

Living longer wouldn't be desirable unless you stayed bright-eyed, on your toes, and free of disease throughout those extra years.

Consider eyesight, for example. By about age fifty-five most people cannot "accommodate" very well. That is, they cannot read newsprint if it's held, say, a foot away from their eyes. The print blurs and they have to hold the paper farther away to bring the print into sharp focus. The lens of the eye stiffens with age, and the eye muscles can no longer make it thinner or fatter in response to what you are trying to see.

If you start the Anti-Aging Plan with caloric limitation well before the stiffening of the lens, the time of accommodation failure will arrive much later in life. The same holds for cataract development.

Athletic ability is a reasonably good marker of functional age. You can't persuade a mouse to play tennis but you can measure its muscular and motor coordination by a sort of log-rolling test. Place the mouse on a rod about the thickness of a broom handle, which is held four feet off the floor and rotated slowly at a fixed speed. Not liking to fall from that height, the mouse will try to stay on the rod. The observer records how many times the mouse falls off in six one-minute trials. In this simple but very good test of a mouse's "athletic ability," the 32-month-old nutrient-rich, calorie-limited mice did just as well as 12-month-old ad lib-fed mice, and far better than 32-month-old ad lib-fed mice, who in fact fell off most of the time. Thirty-two months is quite old for a mouse, yet calorie restriction kept them functionally young.

In terms of the Biospherian experience, we may note as a kind of testimonial that I was the oldest Biospherian at age 69. The others ranged from 31 to 42. Yet having been on the Anti-Aging Plan for five years before entry, I was able to sustain the enormous physical stress of the two-year experiment right alongside the others who were thirty to forty years younger.

In many sports enjoyed by humans an older person can train up to nearly the ability of a much younger person, but let's look at a sporting event in which older humans cannot do this: running the New York Marathon. The fastest recorded times in relation to age are shown in the solid-lined curve of Figure 2.2. Judging by animal data measuring overall physical fitness and performance extrapolated to human performance, in a human population on the Anti-Aging Plan with calorie limitation for a substantial period of years, the curve should appear as shown by the dotted line. This is a remarkable showing! To sustain this much energy output, the older Anti-Aging Plan calorie-limited runners would doubtless need to refeed and gain some weight well before the race, but they would be physiologically much younger than their chronological age.

The China Health Project

A massive recent study of food patterns in relation to disease among 6,500 (largely rural) Chinese followed from 1983 until 1990 — a study undertaken by a consortium of Cornell University, Oxford University, and Chinese scientists (called the China Health Project) — adds a great deal to our knowledge about nutrition and health.

The Chinese consume 20 percent more calories than Americans but are 20 percent thinner. Their diet includes only half as much calcium as ours (they eat hardly any dairy products), yet they are at a much lower risk for osteoporosis. Their average intake of fiber runs as high as 77 grams in some regions, more than twice the 35 grams recommended in the United States, but there is no evidence of the impaired mineral absorption American nutritionists warn about if fiber intake is excessive. The Chinese diet derives only 15 percent of its calories from fat, compared to the 35 to 40 percent in the United States. Seventy-seven percent of their calories come from complex carbohydrates; in the United States the figure stands at only 45 percent, half of these from simple sugars. Finally, the Chinese consume a third less protein than Americans do, and only one tenth as much protein from animal foods.

What do these dietary differences translate to in terms of health? For Chinese men average blood cholesterol is about 138; for American men, it is 212 (with range of 155 to 274). Death from heart disease among the Chinese is only 6 percent of the U.S. incidence; breast cancer occurs at one-fifth the U.S. rate; colon cancer, at about one-third the U.S. rate.

There is no limitation of calories, but the "quality" of the Chinese diet is excellent and health-promoting. While not selected by computer techniques to approach RDA amounts in all essential nutrients — as the Anti-Aging Plan is — the overall food pattern resembles that of the eight inhabitants of Biosphere 2, and *their* diet, the Biospherian diet, is a modification of the Anti-Aging Plan with calorie limitation.

Important features of the Chinese diet, of the diet of Biosphere 2, and the "average" Western diet are shown in Table 2.2. While certain differences exist between our Anti-Aging Plan and the Chinese diet, the findings regarding the China Health Project, the scientific evidence of the Biospherian experiment, and the vast amount of animal evidence behind the formulation of the Anti-Aging Plan — while set up quite independently — are mutually reinforcing. All signs point in the same direction. Our recommendations are on solid ground.

Table 2.2. COMPARISON OF THE NUTRIENT MAKEUP OF THE TYPICAL CHINESE DIET, THE BIOSPHERE 2 VERSION OF THE ANTI-AGING PLAN, AND THE TYPICAL WESTERN DIET.

Nutrient	China	Biosphere 2	West
Total protein (g/day)	64	63	91
Plant protein (g/day)	60	53	27
Carbohydrate (g/day)	524	353	243
Fat (g/day)	43	20	114
% of calories from fat	15	10	43
Total calories/day	2,636	1,860	2,360
Dietary fiber (g/day)	45	55	10

Chapter 3

The Caloric Limitation Principle

Ｗe see from Figure 3.1 that the average life span of the citizens of ancient Rome was about 22 years. Disease, war, famine, and other calamities carried them off at this early average age. As the centuries went by, conditions improved; the average life span increased to about 50 years by 1900. Today it stands at about 75 years from time of

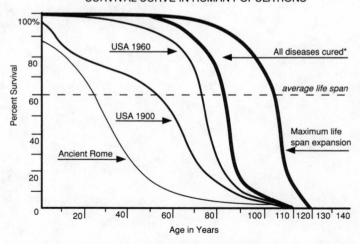

SURVIVAL CURVE IN HUMAN POPULATIONS

Figure 3.1 Survival curves in human populations: ancient Rome, USA 1900, USA 1960, the *curve resulting if most of all diseases were cured but the basic aging process still continues, and a curve representing maximum life span extension.

birth, depending on what (Western) country you are in. But notice: The curves for ancient Rome, U.S.A. 1900, and U.S.A. 1960 (the same for today) all terminate at about 110 years. Under all conditions encountered in history so far, 110 years represents the maximum life span, determined by genetic (hereditary) factors inherent in each species.

We don't know why yet, but each species has a different maximum life span: mice and rats, for example, about 3 years, chimpanzees 45 years, and so on. We could draw a different set of curves for each species, but the same rules would apply.

So long as the basic aging process is not influenced, all that humankind can expect in terms of survival from the complete cure of all diseases, is to approach nearer to that fixed 110-year point. Very old people (100 to 110) tend to die not so much from major diseases like cancer or heart disease, but simply don't recover from what for a younger person would be a minor physiologic insult. They literally wear out before 110 is reached. So in that sense we are *close to the end of medical progress on a population basis*, although not of course on an individual basis. "Individual basis" means the point where you personally will fall off society's survival curve.

If you are on the Anti-Aging Plan but simply eat as much as you want, you'll be much healthier and freer of disease. You'll also enjoy a longer average life. But you won't substantially extend your maximum potential life span. You'll still wear out before reaching 110.

If on the other hand, you limit your calories by 5, 10, or 20 percent, you will proportionately project yourself onto a longer maximum life span curve. Depending on when you start, you may live to be 120 with moderate limitation. With a more steadfast limiting of total calorie intake, you may well live 140 years. And your health will be even better, your resistance to disease even greater.

This is one of the great promises of the anti-aging medical diet, the Anti-Aging Plan.

1935: The First Studies, and Where It Went From There

In 1935 Professor Clyde McCay of Cornell University showed that animals on a low-calorie diet far outlived animals allowed to eat as much as they wanted. Clyde McCay also found that the development

of a wide variety of cancers was inhibited by calorie limitation, and beneficial effects on vascular and kidney diseases also accrued. His studies have been confirmed many times, in many top university laboratories, and in a wide variety of animal species. Figure 3.2 from studies in my University of California Medical School laboratory on mice, and from an investigation conducted by Dr. Morris Ross in rats, graphically illustrates this life extension effect.

Starting at any age, the vertical bars (lower half of figure) show *remaining life expectancy* for calorie-limited animals and for animals allowed to eat as much they liked. Take a good look; this is remarkable data. Those animals represented by the first bar — the 0 to 100 days old bar — could expect to live another 625 days if allowed free access to food, but 1,125 days if on that earlier, rodent version of the Anti-Aging Plan. And when all the overfed animals had died, the remaining, dieting animals still had a life expectancy of 320 days. And they didn't actually cross the finish line until 1,800 days.

Human average life expectancy may improve through exercise, antioxidants, and supplements like vitamin E and selenium, but these measures won't budge that finish point of 110 years.

Caloric limitation will almost certainly do so. Those marvelous 1,800-day-old rats would translate into 170-to-180-year-old humans — humans who were functionally young and vigorous throughout most of that life span. *We emphasize, however, that it would be inadvisable for humans to aim for this highest potential — to 170 or 180 years — because this would require starting from earliest childhood. Rats and mice placed on a calorically restricted diet from the outset do achieve the longest life spans, but their adult size is only about two thirds that of unrestricted animals. We don't want to produce a race of four-foot-high humans here. The Anti-Aging Plan should not be implemented until a human subject has achieved full physical maturity and growth.*

Historical Phases

There have been three historical phases in the development of what we now call the Anti-Aging Plan. The first phase was initiated by McCay as noted above. The second was initiated by me in the early 1970s, and dealt with the effects of nutrient-rich caloric limitation on the physiology of the body. How does it affect the immune system, the levels of various hormones in the body, the biochemistry of the body, and things like learning ability, the connective tissue (whose aging leads to wrinkling of skin), and strength and vitality? This and other work, at UCLA and elsewhere, was amplified through the years to show that virtually every age-related function, and resistance to the major diseases — heart disease, cancer, diabetes, kidney disease, mental deterioration, and the general fragility of age — are positively influenced by caloric limitation. General health is at all ages greatly improved. Animals on the diet are more vigorous, look and behave younger. And this applies not just to rodents, but to one-celled organisms, spiders, worms, fish — indeed, throughout the animal kingdom. It would be extremely surprising if it didn't apply to humans as well. Ongoing work at the University of Wisconsin suggests applicability to monkeys, which are primates very similar to humans. And the Biosphere 2 experiments lend direct support to human applicability.

The third phase, presently a major interest as yet unsolved, is the search for mechanisms. What does caloric limitation coupled with nutrient enrichment actually do that brings about all these "global" changes, these far-reaching and inclusive benefits? The answer is not clear, in part because calorie restriction seems to fit every major theory of aging. It increases the body's ability to repair injury to its own DNA (DNA-repair theory of aging), keeps the immune system "younger" longer (immunologic theory of aging), and increases the body's own production of antioxidants or free radical scavengers (free radical theory of aging).

The Anti-Aging Plan Is Absolutely Not A Starvation Diet

Starvation, by definition, is fatal to any species of animal. Caloric limitation should to lead to a weight loss no greater than about 10 percent for women and 18 percent for men over the first six-month period. Due to individual variation in calorie needs in humans, it is not possible to tie a specific calorie level to a certain level of weight loss. It is known for example that one 120-pound woman may maintain her weight with 1,800 calories per day; another may require 2,400. You should judge therefore by weight loss, and adjust your calorie content accordingly.

With animals, when food intake is persistently less than half that of wholly unrestricted animals, you get into actual starvation and the population will slowly die off.   Up to that point, however, or at milder degrees of restriction, there is still a steady increase in life span, retention of youth and vigor, and increased resistance to disease.   So you can restrict at any level you want in the nutrient-rich Anti-Aging Diet's range and still expect substantial benefits in health and longevity.

To avoid any confusion, let us say that 20 percent restriction means that you are still eating 80 percent of what you would be eating under your usual circumstances.   Any greater restriction may have dangerous adverse effects on your health and is not recommended, and 20 percent is only safe if you are very careful about quality food.

Biosphere 2

Near Tucson, Arizona, the experiment known as Biosphere 2 began on September 26, 1991, when the door was shut on the eight human subjects referred to as the Biospherians. I was one of the eight and the physician.   We entered a massive but totally closed ecological space containing rain forest, ocean, savannah, and desert biomes, an agricultural space, and comfortable living quarters.   We lived and worked there for two years, emerging on September 26, 1993.   Our diet, although extremely wholesome, was limited to about 1,800 calories per person per day for the first five to six months, gradually increasing to 2,200 calories per day by the end of the two year period.[1]

During the first eight months inside the Biosphere we underwent gradual but quite substantial weight loss.   The average loss was 18 percent for the men, 10 percent for the women.   In pounds this averaged thirty-three for the men and seventeen for the women.   Despite the gradual increase in calorie consumption, the Biospherian weights stabilized at these lower levels.   Body fat content was 6 to 10 percent for the men, 10 to 15 percent for the women.   These low levels should not be exceeded.   Body fat content can be estimated by measuring skinfold

---

[1] For a complete nutritional and health analysis of the Biospherians, see R. L. Walford and S. Harris, "The calorically restricted, low-fat, nutrient-dense diet in Biosphere 2 significantly lowers fasting blood sugar, total white cell count, cholesterol, blood pressure, and other physiologic parameters in humans." Published in *Proceedings of the National Sciences* in December 1992.   In Biosphere 2 food choices were made and recorded with our nutrition software, the Interactive Diet Planner (see Appendix).

thickness. Fairly good and inexpensive devices are available for doing this,[2] but values below 10 percent for men and 15 percent for women should be checked by your doctor.

Despite dramatic weight loss, the Biospherians did not feel undue hunger, even though we had to do substantial physical labor to keep Biosphere 2 operational. Hunger is less if food quality is better, at any calorie level. We shall see that this applies outside as well as inside the Biosphere.

The health indices of the Biospherians were very positively affected by their low-calorie, nutrient-rich diet. As we have noted, there was a marked decrease in our average blood pressures. An additional reduction in fasting blood sugar values occurred, from preentry averages of 94 for men and 90 for women to sustained lower values of 65 for men and 68 for women. These changes parallel those demonstrated in animals whose health and longevity have responded favorably to low-calorie, nutrient-rich dietary regimens.

The sustained drop in blood sugar is particularly impressive, as one of the main current theories about aging and health in later years relates to bodily damage inflicted by high blood sugar levels.[3] High blood glucose levels combine with proteins and DNA and immobolize these critical factors. The chemical reactions clog up essential metabolic reactions. A lowering of blood sugar to the degree observed in the Biospherians has not heretofore been achieved by any other dietary or medicinal regime. This lowering, combined with the other factors noted above, parallel data seen in animals on life-extending diets, and constitute — along with similar changes demonstrated in monkey populations — strong indications that the other benefits so well documented in animal populations would also occur in humans.

Key Points of the Anti-Aging Plan
A key point, which we have just illustrated from the Biospherian experience, is that hunger is less if food quality is better, at any calorie level. The Anti-Aging Plan provides you with as close to 100 percent

[2] We recommend Fat-O-Meter, about $10, available from Creative Engineering, Inc., 5148 Saddle Ridge Road, Plymouth, MI 48170.
[3] A. Cerami, et al., Glucose and aging. *Scientific American* 256 (1987): 90.

or more of the **Recommended Daily Allowance (RDA)** of all essential and important nutritional items as possible, and on a fairly low calorie intake! The food combinations are selected so that every calorie comes from a highly nutritional source, and can be thought of as nutrition packed, a "nutrient-rich calorie." Were this not so, gradual long-term weight loss by calorie restriction, whether for Biospherians or for you, might result in deficiencies in essential nutrients. That clearly would not prolong life, but shorten it — which is why people in underdeveloped countries, eating low-calorie diets because of poverty, crop failures, and food shortages, do not live longer. Their intake is not only low in calories but malnourishing.

Nor can you reach your goal by eating a low-calorie but mediocre diet and supplementing it with vitamins and minerals. Too much remains unknown about essential nutrients. Some are doubtless still undiscovered. Untrimmed hamburger on white bread, topped off with a candy bar and a handful of pills will not suffice. Some supplementation may be beneficial, but the basic diet must be as nutrient rich as the Anti-Aging Plan's "nutrient-rich calorie" implies.

While we're at it, let's dispose of another popular fantasy. You can't achieve optimal nutrition by trying to choose what your body "feels" it lacks, as many health faddists suppose. The fallacy of this attractive idea was exposed by an elegant study published in 1974 by Dr. Morris Ross. Four separate populations of rats were set up. One population received a diet of 10 percent protein throughout life; a second, 22 percent protein; a third, 51 percent. The rats of the fourth population were allowed to select what they wanted from among these three diets. The rats of this fourth group instinctively selected ration mixes that optimized growth and development. They grew faster, reached sexual maturity sooner, and got ultimately heavier than the other three groups. However, and here's what made the experiment fascinating: they experienced *a far higher incidence of tumors and other diseases of aging.*

So you can't just go by what you "feel" that you need in the way of food. After all, children may "feel" they need candy, because they crave it. Parents often think they must pump "energy" into their children to promote growth, and they do it in the form of, say, sugar-packed cookies. That's a serious fallacy. Nature has in part shaped our appetite toward food cravings that promote rapid growth and early sexual maturity, which promotes species survival rather than individual long life. The Anti-Aging Plan promotes *individual* long life, by fueling you only with nutrient-rich energy.

Besides its special application to increasing longevity, you can use the Anti-Aging Plan for an ordinary weight loss program, and it will assure you the best possible nutrition. Most of the popular published diets are in fact deficient in a number of essential nutrients; some are disastrously deficient.

Calorie Intake Is the Key

An essential point of the Anti-Aging Diet is that its *longevity* effect is related solely to weight loss achieved by calorie restriction. Any other method — exercise or any other way to "burn off" calories — won't extend maximum life span. Those slender athletes making the big bicycle race, the "grand tour" every year in France, for example, or performing in yearly competitions, and doggedly training for them most of the rest of the time, may be very healthy today but they won't extend their maximum life spans by burning off calories. In fact, excess energy turnover may exert an opposite effect, may even slightly increase the aging rate, even though it is health-promoting in terms of resistance to certain diseases like arteriosclerosis.

How Many Calories Daily?

The actual calorie intake needed to maintain your present weight depends very much on your hereditary endowment and your childhood food habits. People of the same weight, height, sex, and body build differ substantially in how many calories they need just to preserve their present weight.

Shortly after World War II, University of Minnesota scientists put thirty-two young male volunteers on a 1,600-calorie-per-day diet for six months. Not a nutrient-rich diet, but a nutritionally poor diet, it was tailored to mimic the restricted food combinations available to much of Europe's population after the devastating war. The volunteers lost weight but they leveled off at about 75 percent of their original weight.

The experience of the eight persons who lived inside Biosphere 2 also sheds light on this question. Due to various factors, including some limitation of space available for farming, low light levels, and early-on problems with insect pests, the daily food supply per Biospherian for the first five to six months was, as we have mentioned, about 1,800 calories. However, the available food was extremely wholesome and nutrient-rich — mainly vegetables, grains, legumes, fruit, lots of sweet or white potatoes, a little goat milk (made into yogurt), about two eggs per person per week, and chicken, red meat (goat or pork), or fish once per week. In short, nutrient-rich calories! But two months after entering Biosphere 2, all Biospherians had lost somewhere between three and twenty pounds, and a great deal more after six months.

Judging by our personal experience as well as that of others who have followed the Anti-Aging Plan, and supported by careful monitoring of the Biospherian experience during my two-year stay there, you should start your program with 1,800 calories per day. If that level induces gradual weight loss and improves your sense of health and well-being, you may choose to simply carry on. If you are losing weight too fast, too slowly, or not at all, adjust the level of intake accordingly. Unless advised otherwise by your doctor, the upper level should be 2,200 calories per day. However, we will address the calorie level more fully in Chapter 6.

If You Choose Calorie Limitation
on the Anti-Aging Plan, Will You Be Hungry?

No, at least not for long. After a fairly brief period of adaptation, you won't feel particularly hungry. Why? Because you are eating "nutrient-rich calories." These are characteristically found in foods that are the bulkiest possible low-calorie foods, so that they literally "fill your stomach" better than ordinary combinations. They also contain more nutrients per calorie than most foods. This may contribute to the fact that a diet rich in them is, in the long term, satisfying at a lower average calorie level.

A study at the University of Alabama showed that humans allowed to eat as much as they liked, but only high-quality, wholesome foods, were satisfied with as little as 1,500 calories per day.[4]   However, given

---

[4] Ko Ho Duncan, et al, *Am. J. Clinical Nutrition* 37 (1983): 763.

refined and processed foods, *these same persons* required up to 3,000 calories to feel satisfied. The wholesome foods included fruit, hot cereals, skim milk, soups, salads, pasta, fish, chicken, brown rice, vegetables, and whole-wheat toast and rolls. The "refined" foods were bacon, eggs, juice, buttered toast, fast and fried foods, steak, buttered vegetables, whole milk, cake, and ice cream.

A study done recently at the University of Minnesota further illustrates the point. Breakfasts of orange juice and a cold cereal with milk were fed to five groups of healthy adults. Each group was given one of five cereals containing various amounts of fiber: Post Toasties (zero fiber content per 100 grams of cereal); Shredded Wheat (11 grams per 100); Bran Chex (18 grams per 100); All Bran (35 grams per 100); and Fiber One (39 grams per 100). The group given the highest-fiber cereal at breakfast consumed an average of 150 calories less per day than those on the lowest fiber cereal.

The Biospherian experience corresponds exactly to these observations. Despite at least three hours per day of heavy physical labor, mainly intensive farming, the Biospherians on their 1800-calorie-per-day intake were not overly hungry.

You'll consume far fewer calories and feel completely satisfied if you simply eat a nutrient-rich, high quality diet — the Anti-Aging Plan for example — but eating as much of it as you want. A modest restriction from that level will lead to slow weight loss, and won't leave you feeling famished.

Must You Give Up All the Nutrient-Poor Things You Like to Eat?

Cake and ice cream, lemon meringue pie, pecan pie (about the highest combination of fat and sugar in anybody's cookbook), hamburgers, doughnuts, whipped cream, and so on: Must all of these be avoided at all costs? Well, certainly you must cut down on them. But the Anti-Aging Plan is a long-term affair. So the answer is a cautious "No, but be within reason." An occasional indulgence won't matter. And as you get into the diet, your desire for such foods will wither.

Consider vegetarians. They do not feel deprived; they just don't eat meat. And you, like vegetarians, will not feel calorie-deprived or low in energy as the quality of your food improves. You'll be getting better eyesight and hearing, too, at every age, a sharper intelligence, more pep, and an increased feeling of well-being.

When to Begin the Anti-Aging Plan

Almost certainly, the sooner you begin, the longer and healthier your life. Just the same, wait until you are fully grown. As we have mentioned, animals placed on a calorically limited diet in early childhood achieve the longest life spans, but their adult size is only about two thirds that of fully fed animals.

If you are in middle age when you begin, you will very substantially improve your overall health, and also increase your life span. The life span extension will of course be even greater i f you start at around age 20.

Advice to Parents

Very clearly, for the reasons given above, you should *not* put your still-growing children on a calorie-restricted diet with the intent of giving them extended life spans. But if you use the principles and recipes given in this book to increase the *quality* of foods served at your family table, with plenty of nutrient-rich food combinations, your children will benefit in two ways: (1) directly, from eating a healthier diet; and (2) indirectly (but throughout the rest of their lives) from becoming accustomed to better food habits. Remember that your appetite, your food "cravings," are to a considerable extent established by your early feeding history— by what is served or allowed at the family table while you are growing up. Set the example at your own table. You can greatly influence what your child will crave to eat for the rest of his or her life. That's a great opportunity, and a great gift for a parent to give!

Why Live a Lot Longer Anyway?

Let's rephrase the question. Do you want to be *functionally* younger longer, middle-aged longer, and "young-old" longer in full possession of your faculties? These are the periods that will be extended by the Anti-Aging Plan, and not the final period of being very old and feeble. That last period remains about the same. Let's say you were born in 1960 and live until 2080 (120 years). The first 100 to 105 years will be years of vitality and well-being, and you will *appear* about thirty years younger than your birthday age.

You'll have to decide for yourself. But be sure that you have the right picture. The extra years are vigorous, disease-free years, not wrinkled and doddering years. You can, if you like, enjoy having two to three professions, real full-blown professions — not the slow slide toward oblivion facing most of today's elderly retired.

A major part of this book is its hundred new and delicious nutrient-rich recipes. And still another is our presentation of a twenty-first century international orientation in the menus. In our quest for nutrient-rich foods and food combinations, we have looked through many of the world's cultures and found treasures in the cuisines of other lands. We also offer nutrient-rich recipes for such simple American classics as hamburgers, pumpkin pie, and chocolate layer cake. Here are the newest and most exciting nutrient-rich combinations (as well as the old standbys but in new combinations) from the earth's bounty.

Human Lifespan and Other Beneficial Effects

It has been shown beyond question in animals that a nutritionally balanced but low-calorie, "nutrient-rich" diet greatly retards aging, increases life span, and reduces the incidence of age-related diseases. Will these impressive benefits occur in humans? In our view the answer is definitely "yes, with a high order of probability." That means, "almost certain." Absolute certainty may not be available for thirty to forty years, since lifespan experiments in humans require many decades. If you wait that long, you'll miss the "almost certain" chance. That's a choice you have to make.

Fortunately, there are less-than-lifetime-long studies that already show the Anti-Aging Plan's effect on disease susceptibility indicators, and on various physiological aspects of aging. These studies include the Biospherian experiment. Measurable changes in humans on a low-calorie, nutrient-rich diet parallel those reported for animals.

Other Studies in Humans:
The Okinawans of Japan

A number of isolated populations exist that are reputed to contain exceedingly long lived people: the Hunzas in the mountains of India, the inhabitants of the high mountain valley of Villcabamba in South America, and in what used to be called Soviet Georgia. None of these population groups are on anything resembling a low-calorie, nutrient-rich diet, and later investigations have failed to confirm their reputed longevities.

The one exception is the population of the islands of Okinawa in Japan. The Okinawans eat mainly fish and vegetables, a high-nutrient, low-calorie diet. The total energy intake of school children in Okinawa is only 62 percent of the "recommended intake" for Japan. The intake of sugar is only 25 percent of the average for Japan; of cereals, 75 percent; of green and yellow vegetables, 300 percent; and of fish, 200 percent. Total protein and lipid intake are about the same as the Japanese average, but total calorie intake is 20 percent less.

In Okinawa the death rates from stroke, cancer, and heart disease are only 59 percent, 69 percent, and 59 percent respectively, of those for the rest of Japan. In the last decade, the total death rate of people 60 to 64 years of age was only 1,280 per 100,000 in Okinawa compared to 2,181 per 100,000 elsewhere in Japan. Accurate legal birth records have been examined and Okinawa has five to forty times the incidence of people over 100 years of age as any other Japanese island. These impressive longevity and health data have been attributed by Japanese scientists to the Okinawans' low-calorie, high-nutrient diet.

Anorexia Nervosa

Anorexia nervosa is an illness usually affecting young people, especially women, who become overly concerned with body image. For psychological reasons, they eat so little they gradually starve. However, they often eat a rather good diet in terms of nutrient *quality*, one egg a day for example, and nothing else. Typically, they restrict their intake of fat and carbohydrate severely but allow themselves relatively more protein in vegetables and low-fat cheeses. Thus, they undergo drastic body weight losses but with considerably less comparative *mal*nutrition than seen in individuals semistarved from famine or poverty. Anorexics do surprisingly well despite their growing emaciation — *for a time.* In the early stages they may even appear superhealthy: hyperenergized, resistant to colds and other infections — and their immune response capacity may actually be increased above normal despite a lower-than-normal white blood cell count. Similar patterns are seen in calorie-limited animals. But eventually, if the anorexia continues and actual starvation dominates the body's machinery, health declines, and death may follow.

The phenomena of *early*-stage anorexia support the concept that calorie restriction leads to physiologic changes in humans similar to those in other mammals.

These conclusions should not persuade anorexics that somehow they are on the right track. They are not! Despite some early-stage overlap in physiologic findings, anorexia nervosa is a life-threatening mental, physical, and emotional disorder that must be treated. Untreated, it can be fatal.

Weight Loss Programs in Humans

Long-term (three-to-nine-month) very low-calorie diets (usually around 400 to 600 calories per day) have been used in the treatment of severe obesity and in diabetes. This level of restriction is much more extreme than the calorie limitation of the Anti-Aging Plan, and would lead to outright starvation if continued indefinitely, but it yields metabolic effects in humans similar to those seen in rodents on the nutrient-rich calorie-limited regimens. These include an improved insulin response and regulation of blood sugar, and an increase in protein synthesis and turnover.

The Biospherians

The eight people inside Biosphere 2 for two years lived for well over six months on an 1800-calorie allotment of the foods resembling the Anti-Aging Plan's combinations. During the first several months at this calorie level, all Biospherians lost a substantial amount of weight, from 14 to as much as 50 pounds, depending on the person. This weight loss was accompanied by a drop in total white blood cell count to below normal values, a drop in fasting blood sugar, in blood pressure and a remarkable drop in blood cholesterol, as we have detailed elsewhere. These physiologic features are hallmark findings in rodents on life-extending calorie-limited regimens.

Evidence for General Health
Enhancement by the Anti-Aging Plan

There is no doubt that the Anti-Aging Plan, even at a very modest level of calorie restriction, will exert great health benefits, whatever effect it has on life span. The general health benefits encompass and extend beyond recommendations by the American Heart Association and the fine work done by Nathan Pritikin and more recently by Dr.

Dean Ornish. Studies by these institutions and individuals concern disease prevention only and have not been extended to retardation of aging.

Evidence on the relation of high fat intake to various cancers rests on comparisons between different countries. Populations with a high fat intake show more cancer, especially of the breast and large bowel, than populations with low fat intakes. However, unless carefully engineered, high fat diets are also higher in calories, and a number of authorities now believe that it is the higher calorie intake of the fat-eating populations that causes most of the difference. This would accord with animal studies in which calorie restriction markedly reduces the incidence of breast cancer. Indeed, in animals in whom breast cancer is being induced by giving them carcinogenic agents, potentiation by a high fat intake can be almost completely overridden by reduction of calories from other sources.

Easy Weight Loss

With little or no effort you will be able to restrict both calorie and fat intake on the Anti-Aging Plan. When people switch from the usual American diet (what is termed in animal studies the cafeteria diet), to a really wholesome diet, but allowed to eat as much as they want, they consume substantially fewer calories. Once again the Biospherian experience corresponds quite closely to this statement. The Biospherians, who performed rigorous physical labor much of the day, adapted to an 1,800-calorie-per day intake of nutrient-rich, wholesome foods, gradually increasing this to 2,200 calories per day, and they were not overly hungry. A well-engineered nutrient-rich diet, containing all the essentials in balanced proportions, leads to satiety on fewer calories than most people eat on a day-to-day basis.

You will gradually lose weight on the Anti-Aging Plan even if you do not consciously limit your calorie intake, because you will naturally eat less. And even a mild restriction beyond your accustomed intake (say 10 percent), will add a few vigorous years to your life, judging from animal studies. Your overall health will be markedly improved, at whatever level of calorie intake you select.

The major purpose of this book is to offer foods and food combinations that are nutrient rich to the highest degree possible while still tasting delicious. This requires a greater variety of foods, herbs, and spices than was available to the Biospherians, while retaining the same basic principles. We have combined state-of-the-art nutritional and gerontological knowledge with computer technology to shape recipes that fulfill all of your nutritional needs in the most calorically economical way possible.

The diet in this book is also designed to take as little time as possible to prepare and to introduce the reader to new and interesting food choices.

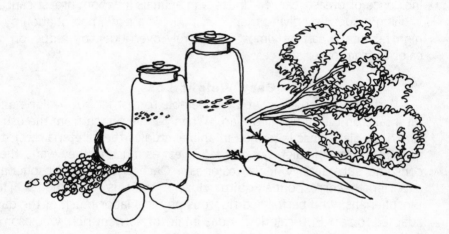

Chapter 4

Health Markers

People tend to accept their daily energy level and their sense of physical decline beginning in middle age as normal and unrelated to diet. "Normal" in this sense means average, it means what is happening to the vast majority, it means acceptance of disability and death in your seventies or eighties, rather than freedom from disease and the enjoyment of an active, vigorous, youthful life to well beyond the century mark. Many people simply have not experienced the increased well-being and remarkable physical transformation that a truly wholesome diet guarantees.

There are tests you can do yourself, or have done by your doctor, which give an indication of your "functional" age and/or your health status. Both types of tests are often referred to as biomarkers. While there is some overlap between biomarkers of "functional" age and those of health, the two categories are not the same.

Biomarkers or indicators of *health status* mainly reflect susceptibility to disease. If you are a relatively sedentary person on a diet high in saturated fats and fairly high in total calories, you are almost certainly developing arteriosclerosis at a rate much higher than active persons on a good diet. This situation can be estimated rather well by certain health indicators, mainly your blood fat profile. But having severe arteriosclerosis, even though it may kill you — from a heart attack or stroke, for example — doesn't necessarily mean you are "functionally" older in your whole body. You may have skin that is unwrinkled and hair that is without graying, but still have blood vessels in your heart that are progressively clogging up. Your blood fat profile will tip you off to this situation while you still have time to effect a change.

Biomarkers of *functional age* are different.   They estimate whether the very fundamental processes of aging are going on within you at the normal rate, or slower, or faster. While individual biomarkers of aging may be measuring the physiologic status of one system, they really reflect the age-status of all systems, of the whole body. They are to be compared with your chronological or birthday age. Are you 50 years old by birthday age but "functionally" 35, 65, or are you right on the norm?

Biomarkers of Health

Basically these are indicators of your susceptibility to disease, principally arteriosclerosis and heart disease, diabetes, kidney disease, and others. Having good biomarkers or health indicator levels of this type will not mean that your maximum potential life span has been extended, or that your fundamental rate of aging has been slowed. But they will indicate that the survival curve of which you are a member has a more rectangular shape (Figure 3.1) so that your *average* life expectancy has been increased.

Health indicators are much easier to influence than those of functional age. A good diet, such as the one given in this book, even without caloric limitation, coupled with exercise, high fiber intake, selected supplements, avoidance of stress and noxious environmental agents, and good health habits (not smoking, not drinking overmuch) will substantially influence these indicators. A low-fat diet, for example, will improve your blood fat pattern and go a long way toward preventing and even reversing arteriosclerosis.

All the health indicators are substantially influenced by the food combinations of the Anti-Aging Plan itself, even if caloric limitation is not a major part of the regimen. They are also influenced by the right kind and amount of exercise, and other general health measures, such as relaxation, meditation, working at what you really enjoy, not driving yourself to exhaustion. Adopt as many of these as you can!

Blood Fat Pattern

The indicators here consist of the levels of your blood cholesterol, high-density lipoproteins (HDL), and low-density lipoproteins (LDL). These should be determined by your doctor before you start the Anti-Aging Plan, then again six months later, and occasionally thereafter, according to his directions. You may expect to see a substantial improvement within the first six months, or even sooner.

Obesity

Obesity itself correlates with cancer, heart disease, and a shortened life span. Despite some past controversy, a recent article in the *Journal of the American Medical Association* clearly showed that thin people live longer, healthier lives. Acquired obesity — over-eating and getting fatter as you grow older — is the worst kind. The genetic tendency towards obesity itself probably means better metabolic efficiency, which in and of itself is good. Thus, being thin or even mildly obese when your "tendency" is toward *considerable* obesity is probably very healthy indeed.

Obesity is of greater health risk if it occurs around the abdomen. Such obesity correlates with low HDL concentrations. Fat distributed about the abdomen is called "above the belt" obesity. If that's your type, it is itself a strong risk factor for arteriosclerosis and adult-type diabetes. All you need is a tape measure to make an assessment.

Measure your waistline and then your hips. Then divide the hip measurement by your abdominal girth. This will give you your waist/hip ratio. If the result is 1.8 or greater for a woman or 1.1 or greater for a man, this indicates that you have a cardiovascular risk.

Blood Pressure, Heart Rate, and VO2 Max.

These measure heart function, physical fitness, and resistance to several diseases. Probably they have little to do with your basic aging rate, but they are well worth doing as part of your overall health program. Exercise will also exert a very major influence on all these health indicators.

The systolic blood pressure increases with age from an average value of 120 at about 30 years to 140 by age 80. The increase is linear. A blood pressure of 140/90 at any age represents a lower rung of "high blood pressure." You want to stay below these values. The remarkable fall in blood pressure in the eight people in Biosphere 2 was detailed in Chapter 2.

Heart rate is another parameter influenced by physical fitness. The average normal rate is seventy-two beats per minute but, of course, this may vary widely. A physically fit person, of any age, is apt to have a rate of about sixty or even lower. Biosphere 2 heart rates were generally sixty or below throughout most of our two-year stay.

The VO2 max., or "maximum oxygen consumption," represents the ability of your heart and cardiovascular system to respond to stress. It declines with age and/or poor physical fitness, reflecting a lower maximal attainable heart rate plus a lower capacity of the tissues to extract oxygen quickly from the blood. To measure it, your doctor will have you exercise vigorously on a treadmill or stationary bicycle, and measure the amount of oxygen you consume per minute. Dividing this by your body weight yields the VO2 max.

For middle-aged sedentary men, the average VO2 max. is about 45 ml. of oxygen per minute for every 2.4 pounds of body weight; for men of the same age who are on a good exercise program, the value may be about 58; for world-class athletes, it's about 75.

Biomarkers of Aging

These are less well defined, and they indicate health status less clearly, than the above indicators. At first look, many age biomarkers do in fact *seem* to reflect "functional" age, when taken as averages within populations. Suppose you have two populations of mice, one on nutrient-rich caloric restriction and one on an average-calorie diet. We know these populations will age at substantially different rates. These rates will be reflected in the all-important survival curves and the maximum life spans reached. The hormone levels, blood fat status, condition of the connective tissue, athletic ability, and many other measurable parameters will vary widely between the two populations. The average of each item being measured in the calorically-restricted group will correspond to the values of chronologically younger mice. That will look quite good.

Yet looking more closely, we shall see that *within* each population there will still be a spread: The level of a particular hormone will not be exactly the same for all restricted mice. And some mice will die sooner, some much later, within each population. You cannot use most of these biomarkers — which look so good on a population basis — to predict with any accuracy whether one mouse will live longer than another within the same population. It simply does not correlate as neatly as we might expect. In short, many age biomarkers don't have *predictive* value for how long the rest of the life span is going to be. A significant factor in this situation, of course, is the overlay of disease and its effect on individual survival.

However, a good age biomarker should not be greatly influenced by any environmental situation unless that situation itself is known to influence the rate of aging. The only environmental situation proven to do that is caloric limitation. Thus, *some*, but not all (since health indicators are also influenced by caloric restriction), biomarkerlike changes associated with caloric restriction may be biomarkers of functional age.

These are all scientific questions that cannot be wholly resolved by existing data. But we can assess your functional age fairly well by means of the biomarkers that follow. They have been selected from a much larger list, and they do have some predictive value (where indicated).

Forced Vital Capacity

Probably the best age biomarker now available for humans is the measurement of lung function called forced vital capacity. This represents the amount of air that can be taken in and breathed out rapidly in one very deep breath. This vital capacity, or VC, reflects a complex function, namely, the integrity of the whole respiratory system: the chest muscles and diaphragm, the central nervous system control mechanisms, the elasticity of the lungs. Your doctor can measure your VC on an instrument called a spirometer. VC declines about 40 percent and in a linear fashion, between youth and 70 years of age.

VC has proven the best single predictor of subsequent life span in

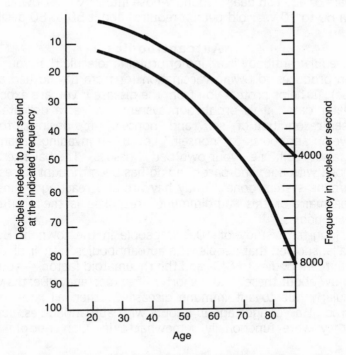

Figure 4.1 Auditory threshold in decibels in relaton to age in women, at sound frequencies of 4000 and 8000 cycles per second (adapted from J.F. Corse, in *Lectures on Gerontology, Vol. 1, part B., Biology of Aging*, ed. A.Vidik [New York: Academic Press, 1982], p. 441).

the large, famous, and still ongoing study involving most of the entire population of Framingham, Massachusetts. The Framingham population has been closely monitored for over forty years, to see how obesity, cholesterol levels, diet, exercise, and other factors affect the incidence of later diseases, especially heart disease.[5]   Individuals with a low VC for their age did not live as long on average as people with high VCs. Furthermore, there was no correlation to whether the individuals were athletic or largely sedentary. This suggests that the VC is independent of this one major environmental influence, and that it may be measuring basic aging, not, for example, an exercise effect.

The hearing threshold has a mild predictive value for later life expectancy in humans. Hearing ability begins to decline at about age 30. The hearing threshold at a fixed frequency is a good way of measuring this decline. How loud must a sound be at a fixed vibration frequency for you to be able to hear it? The concept and the decline are illustrated in Figure 4.1. At 8,000 cycles per second, a person of about 20 years of age can hear a sound whose intensity is as low as 18 decibels; a 60 to 70 year-old person requires about 50 to 80 decibels.

Autoantibodies

A regular antibody is a kind of protein molecule that your immune system produces following vaccination (or from having had an actual disease). It helps protect you from the disease if you are exposed to it at a later date. This production system involves a delicate balance between recognition of "self" and "nonself." It's desirable to be able to develop antibodies to "nonself," i.e., to an invading organism, but not against "self," i.e., your own bodily tissues. The balance becomes disturbed with age, and part of aging has been thought to result from an immune system gone slightly haywire and reacting against "self." The hallmark of this "autoimmune" response is the production of "autoantibodies."

A long-term study of 10,000 people in the town of Busselton, Australia, showed that people with autoantibodies in their blood (especially autoantibodies to DNA and the rheumatoid factor — your doctor will know about these) had a shorter life expectancy. Deaths were not particularly due to autoimmune diseases; rather, all late-life disease occurred at a younger age in people with autoantibodies, suggesting that they were functionally somewhat older than people without

[5] H.W. Hubert, *Circulation* 67(1983): 968

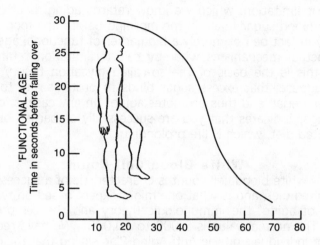

Figure 4.2   Static balance as biomarker of age. Stand on a hard surface (not on a rug) with both feet together, close your eyes, and lift your foot about 6 inches off the ground, bending your knee at about a 45-degree angle. How many seconds can you stand this way before you have to open your eyes? Score = average of three trials.

autoantibodies in their blood. So ask your doctor to test your blood for the presence of autoantibodies — particularly since caloric limitation has been shown to exert a markedly beneficial effect on these phenomena. It knocks autoimmunity for a loop!

Static Balance
This is one test you can do on yourself. How long can you stand on one leg with your eyes closed without falling over? A person 20 or younger can do so more or less indefinitely; an 80-year-old person, not at all. The decline is thus very steep, as illustrated in Figure 4.2. Unfortunately, this test has never been applied in a large predictive population study, so its ultimate value as a functional age biomarker is uncertain. However, because it involves very complex functional parameters indeed, it remains the best candidate for a biomarker you can do yourself. If you can balance for ten seconds, you are functionally 50 years old or less; twenty-five seconds, 30 years old or less.

Fasting Blood Sugar

Caloric limitation, which we know retards aging, is characterized by a low blood sugar taken in the morning before any food ingestion. This may in fact be not merely a biomarker of functional age, but one of the actual mechanisms whereby calorie limitation retards aging. Indeed, this is the basis of the so-called glycation theory of aging, which suggests that excess sugar binds to proteins and to the DNA genetic material, and thus promotes aging. In any case, a low fasting blood sugar indicates that you are successfully embarked on a calorically limited diet, which is life prolonging.

White Blood Cell Count

A low white blood cell count is characteristic of a successful calorically limited diet, and is what one might expect based on two current theories of aging, the immunologic theory and the cell-proliferation theory. The normal value is 5,000 to 10,000. We have received letters from individuals on the Anti-Aging Plan saying that their doctor is concerned that their white blood cell count is below 5,000, for example 4,000. He is right to be concerned. A low and falling white blood cell count may *in some instances* indicate serious disease. But not always. Mice on a calorie-limited diet have very low white blood cell counts, but are extremely healthy. We see from Table 4.1 that the Biosphere 2 inhabitants' white blood cell count was on the average at the lowest limit of normal, and some well below that limit. Thus, a low white blood cell count, like low blood sugar, is a good indicator that you are successfully carrying out a calorie-limited diet. You must, however, let your doctor make sure it does not reflect some problem unrelated to caloric limitation.

Definitely do the static balance test. Have your doctor do a fasting blood sugar, white blood cell count, and the test for autoantibodies. The static balance test is fun and easy, the next three are necessary baselines, and they are all easy. VC and hearing tests are good but less easy, and their effects are visible only on a very long term basis, so you can wait until you are fully into the diet before running these.

Some Remarkable Biospherian Biomarkers

After six months in the Biosphere, one 150-pound male Biospherian came down to a trim and fit 127. His blood pressure went from 135/90 to a comfortable 100/70. The heaviest man lost fifty pounds. His cholesterol fell from 215 to 129, his blood pressure from 100/70 to 80/50.

Table 4.1 given below, summarizes the degree of weight loss and

Table 4.1 CHANGES IN BIOMARKERS FOLLOWING SIX MONTHS ON ANTI-AGING-TYPE DIET IN BIOSPHERE 2 (adapted from Walford et al., Proceedings of the National Academy of Sciences, 1992)

Month	Body Weight Pre	6 mo.	Blood Sugar Pre	6 mo.	Cholesterol Pre	6 mo.	Blood Pressure Pre	6 mo.
1.	208	158	105	82	215	129	100/70	80/50
2.	148	135	81	77	145	100	100/70	90/60
3.	148	126	89	60	196	107	110/72	70/40
4.	150	127	99	72	190	125	135/90	110/70
5.	165	142	101	69	209	122	110/80	100/60
6.	130	115	77	68	146	83	00/60	80/40
7.	123	111	101	68	231	168	110/80	90/60
8.	116	100	8	73	199	119	110/70	85/50
Avg.	148	126	92	70	191	119	109/77	76/57
% chng.	15%		20%		38%		30%/27%	

	White Blood Cell Count pre.	6 mo.
1.	6,500	4,100
2.	6,400	5,600
3.	7,200	5,700
4.	5,600	4,900
5.	5,600	4,700
6.	7,200	5,000
7.	7,200	5,500
8.	7,800	4,800
average	6,600	5,000
% change	24%	

the remarkable changes in a number of biomarkers and/or health status indicators in the eight people inside Biosphere 2 after six months on their version of the nutrient-rich Anti-Aging Plan. No other long-term sustainable diet has ever been shown to produce changes as dramatic as these. The calorie intake per day for all individuals was 1800 for the first six months. The indicated changes were quite visibly in progress after one to two months. Over the remaining eighteen months, calorie intake rose gradually to 2,200; however, all the weights, biomarkers, and health status indicators remained at about the six-month levels.

Your Doctor's Role

To measure the aforementioned biomarkers, you need a doctor's help. If you don't have one, ask for recommendations from friends. Compile a short list. Then call your county medical society, listed in the telephone book, and ask for the credentials of the physicians on the list. Say you are interested in finding a doctor who is a general practitioner or a specialist in internal medicine. The county medical society will not give a specific recommendation that one doctor is better than another, but they will tell you what medical school each person graduated from, where they served their internship, their residency, what hospitals they are on the staff of, and other matters. If they are on the attending staff of a major hospital in your area, that's a strong plus. Some physicians may be very friendly, affable, good talkers, and have good bedside manners but aren't really top doctors, and so cannot get on a major hospital staff. Major hospital affiliation is not foolproof, but it's a good guide.

Having narrowed your list to a few doctors, call them up, ask their fee schedule, and say you are interested in going on a special diet and want a pre-diet checkup. Be sure to state straightforwardly that this is the purpose of your appointment. If the doctor seems to put little importance on diet as a key factor in superior health, go elsewhere. Today the best doctors know the importance of diet to health. Ideally you want someone with satisfactory medical credentials and an open mind about nutritional preventive medicine. Of course, if you already have a good family physician, go to him or her. If your doctor is interested, you might suggest that he or she read *The 120-Year Diet* (available in paperback from Pocketbooks), in which the scientific background for the Anti-Aging Plan is spelled out in detail. If he wants even more information, suggest the book *The Retardation of Aging and Disease by Dietary Restriction* which I co-authored with Dr. Richard Weindruch (see Appendix D).

Chapter 5

Getting Started

There are two methods for starting the diet. Some people are comfortable with sudden change, others with gradual change. The two different methods for starting the Anti-Aging Plan are geared to these two categories. The first, sudden method we call Rapid Reorientation; the second, slower method we call Gradual Reorientation.

Method 1: Rapid Reorientation

For the first four weeks, do what the eight people in the Biosphere did: Eat only the Anti-Aging Plan nutrient-rich recipes and food combinations for every meal, and limit your daily intake of calories to 1800. This will get you off to a good start, change your eating habits, and, unless you are quite a small person, induce substantial weight loss; but we emphasize that this rapid reorientation method is intended for your first two to four weeks only. Why? Rapid weight loss on a *continued* basis may be too fast for an increase in metabolic efficiency to take place. This increased efficiency is probably responsible in part for the health-enhancing effects of the Anti-Aging Plan, and for the fact that the diet will not leave you hungry.

Animal experiments have shown that gradual weight loss works best. It is your own decision whether you want to eat as many nutrient-rich calories as you wish (and you will still lose weight and be healthier this way, so long as you do not dilute the nutrient-rich calories with nutrient-poor ones), or whether you want to limit your caloric intake enough to retard aging and extend lifespan. The basic idea of the Anti-Aging Plan is similar for both options: Escalate yourself into this genuinely wholesome, scientifically planned diet, which is easy to prepare and to follow, then regulate your calorie intake according to your personal health/longevity goals.

And there is one more reason why we advise you — as a beginner on the Anti-Aging Plan — to follow the Biosphere 2 regimen initially for not longer than four weeks: the eight Biospherians lived in an enclosed world, a controlled environment. You are living in a world where the norm often involves nutrient-poor eating habits. Our aim for you is a success-filled start-up and a relaxed transition. Four weeks at the Biospherian level of caloric limitation is all that you should aim for initially. Then merge into the Anti-Aging Plan without any caloric limitation for a while, until you decide whether you want to practice the diet with or without a percentage of caloric limitation.

Remember two things about the Anti-Aging Plan: (1) It is a proven technique that results in your eating fewer calories, spontaneously and without having to struggle with an unsatisfied appetite; and (2) for this particular effect, and for weight loss and general trimming of your body's contour, it relies on your eating nutrient-rich calories only. You must eat either the recipes we have designed, or your own recipes so long as you have created them with the same criteria we have used. With no limitation on quantity, but with this change in quality (to the Anti-Aging Plan's nutrient-rich foods), you'll still lose weight and feel better. If you add the option of enough calorie limitation to put your weight below your set-point and using the same menus, you may expect to live longer, age somewhat less rapidly, be more resistant to disease, and feel better. If you choose a limitation sufficient to maintain you at 10 to 25 percent below your body's set-point, and follow it carefully, then expect the full rewards of extended youth and substantially retarded aging!

Method 2: Gradual Reorientation

During the first week you eat the Anti-Aging Plan for one day — that is, on that day you choose for one of your meals a One-A-Day Megameal (Chapter 10 offers 30 of these meals to choose from, and Appendix B tells you how you can create your own expanding variety of One-A-Day Megameals). Eat as much of it as you want, and for the rest of the day eat as much as you want of the Free-Choice nutrient-rich recipes and food combinations in Chapter 11. Do the same for two days your second week, three days your third week, and so on, until by the eighth week you are eating on the Anti-Aging Plan full time.

The Basics of the Nutrient-Rich Meal Plan Full Time

You cook on only one day each week. On that day, cook eight servings (assuming that you are cooking only for yourself) of a single One-A-Day Megameal (see Chapter 10 for these One-A-Day Megameal recipes) and freeze seven of them. These One-A-Day Megameals have been engineered by computer techniques to contain from 50 to 60 percent or more of the RDA of all essential nutrients. The recipes have been crafted, refined, and extensively taste-tested. They're of gourmet quality. And they meet all of the criteria of the Anti-Aging Plan: low in calories, low in fat, much better in the "quality" of fats than what most people consume, low in simple sugars and carbohydrates, high in complex carbohydrates, and high in fiber. They have been further designed so they can be readily frozen.

After seven weeks you will have made forty-nine (seven times seven) frozen meals, of seven varieties, each supplying at least half of everything you need on a daily basis. Select one for either lunch or dinner. For the other meals you simply remain generally health conscious, using your own good sense and the specific suggestions we shall make, such as the Free-Choice recipes.

Whether to Limit Your Calories, and By How Much Initially

Going for longevity on the Anti-Aging Plan requires caloric limitation. We advise you to aim only for a level of limitation that you can be comfortable with, and which leads to *gradual* weight loss. For most people (depending on their size) an intake of about 1,800 calories will do this. See how that level works for you, and when you reach your selected new body weight, increase the calorie intake enough to keep you there. Any person *can* physiologically adapt to this level of limitation and experience no physical hunger *provided that nearly every calorie eaten is a nutrient-rich calorie.*

Nevertheless some people simply may not be comfortable with long-term calorie limitation of any degree. If you find that you are one of them, just accept it, and enjoy (1) the increased well-being that you will promptly obtain as you eat only nutrient-rich foods and recipes, and (2) the gradual and moderate weight loss that you will naturally achieve on the Anti-Aging Plan, even if you eat unrestrictedly.

Set-Point

If you choose to add caloric limitation to maximize and extend your healthy years, success depends on deciding what your "set-point" is, then gradually losing weight until you are 5 to 10 percent or as much as 25 percent (not more) below that set-point, and staying at the new weight. This must be achieved on a nutrient-rich diet, detailed in this book.

Your personal set-point is an important piece of information to know about yourself. It refers to what your ordinary or natural weight would be if you just ate your usual, accustomed intake. Hereditary and childhood feeding habits fix a "set-point" for each of us, which is then defended by the body's machinery. Unless you grossly overeat or undereat, you tend to maintain this characteristic weight. It can be well above or below the "average" weight for your body build and sex as determined by insurance company tables. For example, I weighed 145 to 150 pounds during my college years, and I still drift toward that weight if I eat a calorie-unlimited diet. Thus 145 to 150 is my set-point. If you are older and have gained weight gradually throughout your life, you should take as your personal set-point your average weight between the ages of 20 and 30.

Your personal set-point, based on heredity and early food habits, may in fact correspond to being moderately obese, or even very obese. In that case, a sustained 10 to 20 percent weight reduction may still leave you slightly obese. Will this still increase your life span and improve your general health?

The answer is yes. Races of mice that are genetically very obese will, when put on a nutrient-dense calorie-limited diet, enjoy very extended life spans and greatly increased health, even though they are still *moderately* obese. If at your personal set-point you are naturally obese, you don't have to lose weight until you are noticeably thin to benefit from the Anti-Aging Plan. Losing 10 to 18 percent of your weight (the Biosphere 2 averages for women and men respectively) might leave you mildly obese but still below your personal set-point, and would significantly extend your average and maximum life spans.

You may also be quite sure you are below your personal set-point (in some cases very much below) if your body fat content is less than 10 percent for men and 15 percent for women, as discussed in Chapter 3.

How Many Calories Per Day ?

What calorie level should you aim for eventually, for a maintenance level? Many people want exact guidelines, especially when it is a question of amounts and possible limitation of amounts. Perhaps it is human nature to want a reassuring feeling of manageability in the midst of change. We want to know that this or that *precise* amount of calories is definitely all right, not too much (thereby protecting one from obesity), and not too little (thereby protecting one from hunger). This is understandable. But there is no exactitude in the realm of human nutrition. People tend to want a particular calorie level to be specified, like 1,500 per day, or 2,000 per day. There are diet programs that pretend to allow you to estimate your basal calorie needs (what it takes just to keep you alive at rest, i.e., to yield enough energy to support the functioning of your vital organs like liver, heart, brain, etc.), then to add the amount of calories expended in different types of exercise. These diet programs are misguided.

The truth is, your personal body is not an average of a lot of bodies. *Your* "normal" body weight is personal; it is not simply an average of a big group of same-height, same-age people. Great individual variation exists, relating, for example, to metabolic efficiency. Naturally thin people tend to be "burners," i.e., they burn off excess calorie intake as wasted heat. Naturally obese people don't do this so much. Instead, they store the excess calorie intake as fat. This ability of a naturally obese person to store excess calories as fat probably reflects evolutionary advantages in the life of prehistoric humankind, to tide one over during periods of food shortage.

How to Begin

Start with either the Rapid Reorientation Plan or the Gradual Reorientation Plan, as outlined earlier in this chapter, and weigh yourself once a week at the same time in the morning. If you are gradually losing weight, stay at that food intake, using the recipes of the Anti-

Aging Plan. If you are not losing weight and feeling healthier, or are losing weight too fast, adjust the calorie level accordingly, either up or down. Do not go on a crash weight-loss regimen, which will only produce the well-known yo-yo effect (you lose, you regain, you re-lose, you regain, as you have seen Oprah Winfrey, Elizabeth Taylor, and other stars do all too often). A change in food habits alone (to the Anti-Aging Plan) will lead to weight loss and greater health; add caloric limitation to that and you will also slow aging.

Method two — Gradual Reorientation — will direct your food habits toward the nutrient-rich menus given in this book. As that change progresses, take a year to reach your new weight level. Eventually you can also learn how to write your own nutrient-rich menus using the software we've created especially for this purpose (see Appendix B).

Going for Simple Weight Loss and Increased Health

The average American diet is long on quantity and short on quality. From 1910 to today, fat consumption has increased by 25 percent. Forty percent of calories are now derived from fat, with two thirds of this coming from saturated fat. Furthermore, even the unsaturated fats people include in their diets have in many cases been chemically altered, the natural cis-double bonds having been converted by processing into the less healthy or downright unhealthy trans-double bonds (up to 17 percent in some commercial vegetable oils, 47 percent in margarine, and by as much as 58 percent in some vegetable shortenings). The average American diet has shifted substantially from complex carbohydrates to simple sugars, exactly the opposite of what one of the major modern theories of aging would prescribe. In the present century we have increased the fats and sugars in our diet, increased animal and decreased vegetable proteins, greatly decreased cereal and fiber intake, and shifted from natural to processed foods. Now that we are living longer (for other and non-nutritive reasons), this bad diet takes its toll in the degenerative diseases of late life. The role of diet in, for example, cancer is represented in Figure 5.1 for both men and women. Its role in arteriosclerosis, heart disease, and diabetes is even greater.

The Anti-Aging Plan, even without caloric limitation, will substantially diminish your susceptibility to all these maladies.

PREVENT WHAT IS GOING TO KILL YOU

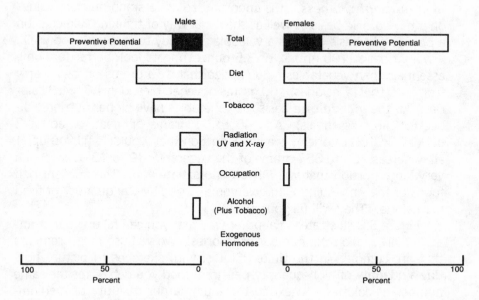

Figure 5.1 Environmental factors and cancer. Only 10-20% of cancers are genetically determined, as shown by the solid portion of the topmost horizontal bar. The rest are due to environmental influences, of which diet is by all odds the most important factor (adapted from G.B. Gori, *Cancer* 43:2151, 1979).

Appetite

Different kinds of foods have quite different amounts of calories per gram or ounce. Butter is a very high calorie-per-gram food. A fresh apple, by contrast, is a low calorie-per-gram food. A vegetable such as cabbage is even lower, and a sweet potato is a medium calorie-per-gram food. What this means is that for the same number of calories, you can eat much larger quantities of some foods than others. High calorie-per-gram foods that are also refined and processed (so-called junk foods) often contain substantial amounts of sugar, and sugar stimulates appetite. People eating these foods, such as hot dogs, cookies, and sweet carbonated drinks, require up to 25 percent more calories to feel satisfied than people on a wholesome diet.

There is no contradiction between *low calories per gram* and *high-nutrient richness*. It is important to understand nutrient values on a *per calorie* basis as well as the usual way of thinking, which is on a *per weight* basis. This is a valuable new way to rate your food. On a weight basis (100 grams, or 3.5 ounces)meats look better for some essentials than vegetables. But notice that 100 grams of meat carry from 140 to 217 calories; 100 grams of vegetables, only 28 to 38 calories. At the *per-calorie* basis the vegetables have higher nutrient values for most essentials. And 46 to 71 grams of meat, or about 2 ounces (= 100 calories), is a small portion that wouldn't fill you up at all, whereas 263 to 357 grams of the vegetables (9 to 13 ounces) is a very large portion that will fill you and satiate you. The nutrient-rich foods of the Anti-Aging Plan give you a large physical quantity of food per calorie. They will fill you up.

Figure 5.2 illustrates in another way that you can fill up your stomach on an economical number of calories! We will use measurements that are common in the United States, with sketches to picture how tiny a quantity of high-quantity-per-gram food you get — for the same number of calories — next to the much larger quantity of medium-calories-per-gram foods, and finally next to the very large quantity of food that you get in the lowest calories-per-gram foods. This should pursuade you and your stomach that you will be fuller, more content, day to day, when you live the Anti-Aging Plan.

This figure has three columns: In the left-hand column are the "high-calorie-per-gram" or "red-light" foods. In the middle column are the medium-calorie-per-gram or "yellow light" foods. In the right-hand column, we put the low-calorie-per-gram or "green light" foods. Notice that refined, processed or junk foods fall into the "red light" column. They are the villains, the worst of the lot.

This figure is entirely *good news*: there are many delicious and nutrient-rich foods that you can eat in *large* quantity, while getting very few calories! During the next week, every time you get an urge for a candy bar, eat a piece of fruit instead. A banana is a good choice. See whether you feel less famished a few hours later than if you had eaten the candy bar.

The Anti-Aging Plan feeds you every kind of food in addition to the kales and broccolis of the vegetable kingdom, at the same time that it

Figure 5.2

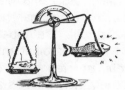

Is Your Diet in Balance?

NUTRIENT DENSITY ON A PER CALORIE BASIS

RED LIGHT FOODS Choose rarely		YELLOW LIGHT FOODS Wholesome foods		GREEN LIGHT FOODS Eat freely	
MORNINGS / 100 CALORIES PER SERVING					
eggs, whole	1 1/4	cooked oats	1/3 cup	egg whites	13 egg whites
English muffin	3/4 of one	cooked Wheatena	1/4 cup	Fiber 1 cereal	3/4 cup
Egg McMuffin	1/3 of one	Pancakes	1	100% Bran cereal	+1/2 cup
w.w. pancakes, mix	1/2 of 1			lowfat cott. cheese	+1/2 cup
(Aunt Jemima)		Nutrigrain, corn	−1/2 cup	lowfat yogurt	+1/2 cup
granola	1 tblsp+1 tsp	millet	−1/4 cup		
		wheat germ	+1/4 cup		
ENTREES / 100 CALORIES PER SERVING					
corned beef	+1 oz	beef sirloin	+2 oz	turnip greens	3/4 lb
lamb chops	+1 oz	chicken w/o skin, roast'd	+2 oz	broccoli	2/3 lb
liver	−1 oz	lamb leg	+2 oz	cabbage	+3/4 lb
chorizo	−1 oz	kidney beans, cooked	2 oz	spinach	3/4 lb
beef-shortribs	+1 oz	potato with skin	1/2	carrots	2/3 lb
CHEESE / 100 CALORIES PER SERVING					
cream cheese	2 tblsp	cottage cheese	+1/3 cup	nonfat cott. cheese	2/3 cup
cheddar cheese	+1 oz	ricotta, part skim	+1/4 cup	lowfat cott. cheese	1/2 cup
reduced fat cheddar	−1 oz	mozzarella, part skim	+1 oz	*(try whipping the above & adding herbs)*	
camembert	+1 oz	feta	+1 oz	mashed swt potato	1/3 of 1 large

− = slightly less, + = slightly more

NUTRIENT DENSITY ON A PER CALORIE BASIS

RED LIGHT FOODS Choose rarely		YELLOW LIGHT FOODS Wholesome foods		GREEN LIGHT FOODS Eat freely	
FATS & OILS　1 oz = 28 grams / 100 CALORIES PER SERVING					
butter	1 tblsp	avocado	2 tblsp	guacamole	1/3 cup
margarine	1 tblsp	Hummus	2 tblsp		
olive oil	2 tsp			unswt apple butter	1/4 cup
sesame oil	2 tsp	chopped olives	2 tblsp	*for baking:*	
canola oil	2 tsp	*for baking:* frozen fruit		over-ripe bananas	2/3 cup
		juice concentrate	1/4 cup	evap. skim milk	1/2 cup
		for sauces: sweet potato	1/3 of 1	*for sauces:*	
				nonfat yogurt	3/4 cup
				potato w/o skin	1/2 of 1
DRESSINGS & SPREADS / 100 CALORIES PER SERVING					
mayonnaise	1 tblsp	Hummus	1 tblsp	catsup	5 tblsp
Miracle Whip Light	1 tsp			mustard	5 tblsp
blue cheese salad drsg	1 tsp	Black Bean Spread	1 tblsp+1tsp	cott. cheese, lowfat	1/3 cup
1000 island salad drsg	1 1/2 tsp	*(see Mushu Chicken recipe page　)*		tofu	1/2 cup
Caesar salad dressing	1 1/2 tsp			nonfat yogurt	1 cup
DESSERTS / 100 CALORIES PER SERVING					
banana cake	1/2" sliver	Maple Angelfood Cake	1 piece	papaya	3/4 of 1
carrot cake	1/2" sliver			Noodle Kugel	2" x 3" piece
cheesecake	1" square	dried apricots	6 large halves		
brownies	1 1" x 2"	raisins	1/4 cup	banana	1 medium
Oreo's	2 cookies	Tropical Dreambars	1 cookie	boysenberries	1 cup
Chocolate Kisses	4 pieces				
pudding + whole milk	1/4 cup	pudding + skim milk	1/3 cup		
BEVERAGES / 100 CALORIES PER SERVING					
martini	1.5 oz	Coca Cola	8 oz	V8 Juice	16 oz
creme de menthe	1 oz	cream soda	6 oz	light beer	12 oz
dessert wine	+2 oz	table wine	5 oz	papaya juice	8 oz
vanilla shake	3 oz	Bloody Mary	4 oz	orange juice	8 oz
Instant Breakfast	3 oz			club soda	as much as you like

− = slightly less, + = slightly more

is calculatedly and pleasurably slanted toward nutrient richness per *calorie*, rather than richness per *weight*, so that your stomach *feels*, and *is*, full! The Anti-Aging Plan includes a large variety of meal plans and food combinations selected both for flavor and *on the basis of their nutrient-rich calorie content, rather than per weight*. Nutrient-rich calories are excellent for your health, your weight, and your satisfied appetite.

Exercise

While exercise is not specifically a part of the Anti-Aging Plan, we are often asked about its effects both on general health and longevity. Here are the answers.

Exercise of the right kind, frequency, and intensity certainly benefits health. It increases cardiovascular fitness, thus decreasing susceptibility to heart attacks and strokes, improves carbohydrate metabolism, delays some of the age-related deterioration of skeletal muscles, and improves brain function.

Exercise promotes a higher level of the beneficial high-density lipoproteins (HDL) in the blood and lowers the level of low-density lipoproteins (LDL). Exercise also benefits the cholesterol/HDL ratio (a better predicator of heart disease than the cholesterol level alone). Male and female joggers, marathon runners, and skiers have very clearly been shown to have an increase in HDL. The beneficial effect of exercise is best achieved by periods (twenty minutes three times per week, for example, will have a measurable effect) of rather vigorous aerobic exercise, in which the pulse rate reaches about 75 percent of the maximum rate for the person's age group. (Maximum pulse rate to reach during exercise can be estimated by subtracting your age from 220, or, better still, by having your doctor do a treadmill test.)

For example: If you are 50 years old, the maximum exercise pulse rate might be 170. Seventy-five percent of that is 128. Your heart rate during twenty minutes of aerobic exercise should be about that for full benefits. Of course, check with your doctor. And you do have to keep it up! If you stop exercising, your blood fat levels will return in a matter of a few weeks to those of a sedentary person.

Besides increasing the insulin sensitivity of the tissues and improving carbohydrate metabolism (both good), exercise retards the slowdown in reaction time that occurs normally with aging. "Reaction time" refers to how many seconds or parts of a second it takes you to react to a stimulus, like a flashing light, or a car that is careening toward you as you cross the street.

Sixty-year-old people who have exercised vigorously for twenty years show reaction times equal to or better than inactive people in their twenties. Not only this, but physically fit individuals display higher levels of so-called fluid intelligence — the ability to think through a problem, as opposed to mere memory.

All to the good, but there are a few aspects of exercise that seem a bit less rosy, at least on theoretical grounds. You should above all avoid the myth that exercise is a sort of universal panacea for health problems, and especially the idea that it's okay to have a high-calorie, even slightly junky diet, as long as you burn off those extra calories by exercise. That's not the case. Animal experiments have clearly shown that exercise may increase the general health but will not increase the maximum life span. The Anti-Aging Plan will of course do both, and to a much greater degree than exercise alone.

Exercise revs up the metabolic machinery, burns more calories, and increases the generation of chemical substances known as "free radicals" in the body. One prominent albeit still controversial theory of aging holds that free radicals are instrumental in aging. If this is true, then exercise has both positive and negative effects. A recent study reported in the *Journal of the American Medical Association* followed 13,344 men and women at various levels of physical fitness, from Level 1 (least fit) to 5 (most fit), over an eight-year period. Those whose treadmill performance placed them in Levels 2 and 3 experienced the lowest death rates over the eight years. Surprisingly, those *very fit* individuals at Levels 4 and 5 did not show a corresponding drop in mortality. Thus, moderate but not excessive exercise appears best from the health standpoint.

The positive health benefits of exercise increase rapidly up to a certain point — corresponding to about fifteen miles of jogging per week (three hours of jogging) — and then plateau out. Therefore, to maximize benefits and keep possible negative aspects to a minimum, we recommend a level of aerobic exercise equivalent to fifteen miles of jogging per week.

If this seems too much for you, twenty minutes three times per week will still do you a great deal of good.

Caution: Just as you should check your health with a doctor before beginning any dietetic changes, you should also check your health before increasing your physical exercise. Then, with your doctor's approval, you should *gradually* begin, or *gradually* increase, your physical exercise.

Chapter 6

Understanding Nutrition

In addition to eating the nutrient-rich meals of the Anti-Aging Plan at least once a day, what rules should guide your eating habits at other times? The following considerations apply whether you eat at home or out.

Your overall intake should be: (1) generally moderate in protein, with emphasis on vegetable as opposed to animal protein sources; (2) low in fat and with an emphasis on "quality" fats; (3) high in fiber; (4) low in simple sugars but rich in complex carbohydrates. We will also recommend certain vitamin and other supplements.

Protein

The amount of "complete" protein a person requires per day is about 0.015 ounces per pound of body weight. This comes to around 2 ounces per day, depending on the size of the person. This amount is required to replace the protein the body loses daily in the form of discarded cells, and proteins broken down or "turned over" through metabolism. Such replacement protein is not used for energy but goes back into the structure of the body. However, at low calorie levels, the body may divert some of this replacement protein into energy use, and leave you relatively deficient in protein for structural use. Thus, on a calorie-limited diet — say below 2,000 calories per day — it is advisable to increase the protein moiety by 10 to 20 percent. You should in fact feel hyperenergized and vital on a calorie-limited, nutrient-rich diet. If, after some months, this feeling of hyperenergy should wane, look first to whether your protein intake is adequate. If not, increase it. Nonfat milk or buttermilk would be a good source for this, since both provide "complete" proteins (see below). If this does not revitalize you, then you are simply at too low a calorie level.

Proteins are made of amino acids. Many of these amino acids can be manufactured by the body itself, but eight cannot and must be obtained from food. These eight are referred to as the "essential" amino acids. When these are present in the daily food intake in the ratios represented by the Recommended Daily Allowance amount, *all* of the ingested protein, i.e., both the essential and the nonessential amino acids, can be used in making the building blocks of the body. If the supply of one essential amino acid is deficient, a portion of the others is merely converted into energy, and burned off. While achieving exact or close to Recommended Daily Allowance ratios is no longer regarded as highly important, it remains of some importance in the Anti-Aging Plan, as you don't want to be burning off extra calories to no benefit. Your caloric needs are best met by complex carbohydrates, not proteins or fats.

Protein intake of the average American has remained fairly constant during the twentieth century, at about 3.7 ounces per day. This is excessive, whatever the calorie level. The concomitant shift in emphasis from vegetable to animal proteins has had additional detrimental effects. Remember: the China Health Project clearly indicated that vegetable proteins are superior to animal proteins in health promotion. Let's consider protein from standpoints both of quantity and quality.

Excess protein intake — the steak and eggs diet, as exemplified, for example, in Dr. Atkin's "Diet Revolution" (a diet that was first published in 1972 and was widely practiced), is unhealthy on a long-term-basis. Experimental studies have shown that such a diet leads to kidney disease and a shortened life span. Furthermore, an increased protein intake, particularly animal protein, speeds excretion of calcium, which may contribute to the development of osteoporosis.

Osteoporosis is one of the major problems of old age. It afflicts 20 million Americans, leads to 190,000 hip fractures per year, and 180,000 "crush fractures" of the spinal column, and it costs $5.3 billion yearly in medical bills alone. Calcium in the diet is thought to help prevent osteoporosis. However, note that osteoporosis is much less common among the Chinese (see Chapter 2), even though their calcium intake is about half of ours. This may well be because their protein is largely of vegetable origin.

Many athletes, especially body builders, have a mania about proteins. They believe that a very high protein intake will increase muscle mass and stamina. That's just not true! There is no direct link between big muscles and big amounts of protein in the diet. Excess proteins are simply metabolized, largely to carbohydrates, or converted into fat and deposited in the abdomen, hips, or elsewhere, and extra energy must to be expended by the body to fuel this metabolism.

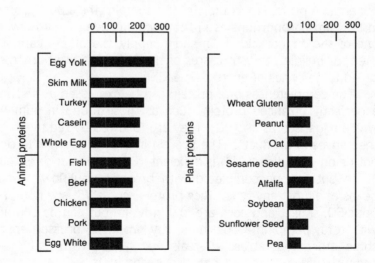

BLOOD CHOLESTEROL (MG/100ML)

Figure 6.1 Effects on blood (plasma) cholesterol levels of feeding various protein preparations to rabbits maintained on cholesterol-free diets (adapted from K.K. Carroll, Federation Proceedings, 41:2792, 1982).

The Anti-Aging Plan seeks to avoid unnecessary energy turnover beyond basic requirements for health, exercise, and pleasure. You don't idle your car with the accelerator halfway down, and you shouldn't be doing the same thing to your body. Only if you are substantially limiting your calories should the proteins be increased beyond the general vicinity of the Recommended Daily Allowance levels (see above).

As to quality, there are advantages and disadvantages to plant as compared to animal proteins. One potential advantage is that plant proteins may tend to lower blood cholesterol and low-density lipoproteins (the LDLs, which are instrumental in producing arteriosclerosis). Figure 6.1 illustrates the effects of proteins from the two sources on cholesterol levels in rabbits. The Chinese experience supports these implications.

On the other hand, it is true that animal proteins are more "complete" than plant proteins in terms of their essential amino acid components. A protein is "complete" if it contains the essential amino acids in the same proportions as in the Recommended Daily Allowances. If one of the amino acids is in short supply, the others cannot be fully used for building the structures of the body, and are burned off in so-called futile cycles of energy expenditure.

The completeness of a protein can be expressed as a score, where a perfectly balanced protein, such as those found in human milk or whole eggs, scores as 100. They are followed by red meat, then fish, then soybean products. The protein in brown rice (white rice should not be on your diet at all!) is deficient in the amino acids isoleucine and lysine but can be completed with broccoli, cauliflower, spinach, or beans of almost any type. Rice protein scores 75, soy flour 70, wheat flour 50. Millet and corn are low in lysine but can be complemented with tofu, pumpkin seeds, nuts, soy products, brussels sprouts, and some other vegetables. Cereals match well with leafy vegetables, peanuts with wheat and oats, soybeans with corn, wheat, and rice. Beans are generally low in methionine and tryptophan, and are well complemented by rice. Achieving 100 percent or more of the Recommended Daily Allowances of the essential amino acids in your diet is easy. To maintain a balanced ratio takes a bit more planning, but it's not something that need become an obsession. Just give it some thought in your selection of daily menus. The food combinations in the

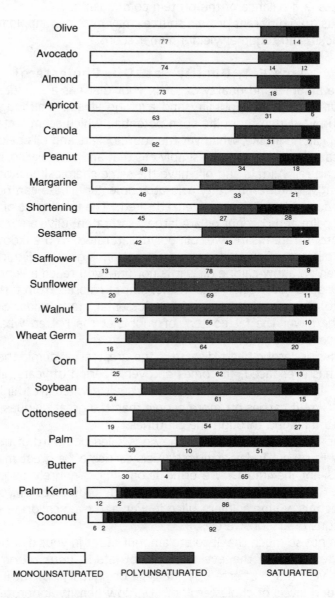

Figure 6.2 Different oils according to their degree of saturation. For example, olive oil consists of a mixture of 77% monounsaturated, 9% polysaturated, and 14% saturated oils.

meal plan and recipes of the Anti-Aging Plan are geared toward completeness and balance of the protein components.

Thus, two different protein sources may mutually supplement what each lacks, and together yield a higher score.

Low Fat, Quality Fat, Oil: Cholesterol

The amount and quality of fat in your diet has a significant effect on your disease susceptibility and average lifespan, although not so much on your maximum life span potential, which seems related *only* to total calorie intake, whatever the source. Fats and oils belong in the same category since fats are simply oils that are naturally solid at room temperature. All fats and oils have the same chemical backbone, glycerol, but with different fatty acid attachments. These can be saturated, monounsaturated, or polyunsaturated. The fatty acids of red meat and of palm and coconut oil are largely saturated; olive and canola oils, monounsaturated; safflower oil, polyunsaturated. A breakdown of different oils according to degree of saturation is given in Figure 6.2.

Even on a low-calorie diet, it is not until you reach a very low level of fat indeed (between 7 and 10 percent of calories from fat) that you run into any potential deficiencies in "essential" fatty acids. So, in general, the lower the fat content of your diet the better, whatever the degree of saturation.

Arteriosclerotic heart disease is the greatest epidemic the Western world has ever faced. It comes on over a period of years, like a slow death. It doesn't look like what we visualize when we think of "epidemic," yet it carries off more people than the great plagues that have afflicted mankind through the centuries.

The Black Death of the Middle Ages killed one third of the population of Europe. Today arteriosclerosis carries off a great many more. But it's not inevitable. We bring it on almost entirely by our eating habits. And unfortunately we start young. Autopsies of young accident victims, young soldiers killed in war, and even children, show definite signs of arteriosclerosis.

It's not so much the absolute amount of fat in your diet that makes the difference, but the level and type of fats *in your blood*, and this level is very much affected by the type or "quality" of fat in the diet. The blood levels of cholesterol, of LDL (low-density lipoproteins), HDL (high-density lipoproteins), and to a lesser extent the triglyceride fats are the important ones.

In the body, cholesterol is packaged into LDL and HDL envelopes for transport to and from the organs. In centrifuged serum, the lipoproteins separate into heavy (high density) and light (low density) types. LDL delivers and HDL removes cholesterol from the tissues. Indeed, HDL has been shown to act as a cholesterol scavenger by removing cholesterol from arteriosclerotic plaques and transporting it (in the form of esters) to the liver, whence it goes into the gallbladder as bile, and then to the gut, where it can be either reabsorbed or excreted. Fiber helps in this excretion. And so, high blood HDL plus a high fiber diet may act together to prevent arteriosclerosis.

If (1) the delivery system is overloaded, and if (2) breaks have occurred in the blood vessel walls (smoking and high blood pressure potentiate such breaks), and particularly if (3) the removal system can't handle the load, cholesterol accumulates in the vessel walls. This leads to progressive arteriosclerosis. Most important in this interaction is the amount of total cholesterol in the blood in relation to the HDL removal system. A ratio of total blood cholesterol to HDL cholesterol of 5 (for example, cholesterol 200, HDL 40) carries an average risk of heart disease; a ratio of 3.5 (cholesterol 200, HDL 57) carries only half the risk. So you want to achieve a low blood cholesterol, high HDL, and low LDL. And *very* low blood cholesterols, such as those reached by the Biospherians (or in fact anything lower than 150), will override and negate the negative influence of a low HDL, if that happens to be your genetic propensity.

Guidelines of the National Cholesterol Education Program give a good estimate of what to shoot for. They include the following: If your blood cholesterol is less than 150, you are very unlikely to have a heart attack regardless of the levels of HDL, LDL, or triglycerides in your blood. Beyond the 150 level, you are still in reasonable shape if your LDL is less than 130, HDL is over 45, and triglycerides less than 150. Besides diet, there is some genetic control of HDL levels, and members of families with persons living to over 100 years of age are often found to have high HDLs — 75 or even higher.

With a few exceptions — and these relate to "quality" of fat — the condition of arteriosclerotic heart disease is lowest in populations eating diets high in complex carbohydrates and low in total fats and cholesterol. The Chinese are a striking example (see Chapter 2). As for the Japanese, they are a modern, high-stress, heavy smoking society, but show a *low* incidence of heart disease — unless they emigrate to the United States and/or adopt American dietary habits (for example, among the Japanese community in Hawaii.)

The traditional Japanese diet is low in fat, particularly in the saturated fats that come from animals and certain products like butter and cheese. However, the modern Japanese diet is rapidly changing. The Japanese have imported some of our bad dietary habits. Fat intake, for example, has increased 300 percent since 1955, contributing to the increase in breast and colon cancer among present-day Japanese.

Vegetarians, like the Hunza tribes of India or the Seventh Day Adventists in America, enjoy a much lower incidence of heart disease than the average American population. Finland, which has the world's highest dietary intake of saturated fats and cholesterol, has the world's highest death rate from heart disease. In the long-ongoing and famous Framingham study in Massachusetts, the risk of heart disease was lowest among those individuals with low blood cholesterol.

These epidemiological studies have been supported by actual experimental studies in humans. In the $150 million study conducted by the National Heart, Lung and Blood Institute, lowering blood cholesterol by a combination of diet and medication clearly reduced the risk of death from heart attacks.

You should make a serious and sustained effort to keep your blood cholesterol below 180, and preferably below 150. Diet and exercise are the keys to this. There is evidence, moreover, that dietary cholesterol has an independent effect on the risk of dying of coronary heart disease over and above its effect on blood cholesterol levels. Based on Western Electric study data, getting 100 mg instead of 300 mg of cholesterol for every 1000 calories eaten means a 47 percent lower risk of fatal heart attack over the next twenty years for a middle-aged man. Table 6.1 gives a brief synopsis of cholesterol and saturated fat contents of representative foods.

TABLE 6.1.
CHOLESTEROL AND SATURATED FAT CONTENT
OF REPRESENTATIVE FOODS

Food plus size of portion	Cholesterol (mg)	% sat. fat
Beef liver (4 oz.)	545	3.0
McDonald's scrambled eggs	399	3.0
Shrimp (4 oz.)	220	0.3
1 large egg	213	2.0
Burger King Whopper w/cheese	113	17.0
Chicken or turkey, skinned (3 1/2 oz.)	95	2.0
Flounder, sole, or clams (4 oz.)	76	0.3
Egg noodles (1 cup.)	50	0.5
Beans, fruit, vegetables	0	0.5

Cholesterol may have up to thirty-two auto-oxidation products, and some of them are quite damaging. Cheeses exposed to air for long periods during processing and then stored at room temperature are likely to contain toxic cholesterol derivatives. It's heat that tends to oxidize the cholesterol in eggs. Fried or hard-boiled eggs are the worst, then scrambled eggs, and soft-boiled eggs are best. It may be less important to limit your egg intake than to eat eggs in as unoxidized a form as possible, i.e., with soft yolks. Any form of powdered egg is especially bad, and many commercially available noodles are made with powdered egg. Avoid them. Oxidation of cholesterol may also take place in powdered whole milk. Powdered skim milk is okay, having no cholesterol anyway; and powdered buttermilk is also acceptable, having very little cholesterol.

Separately from their cholesterol content, the types of fats and oils in your diet are important. Oils high in monounsaturated fatty acids are the best for your health (olive oil, canola oil — see Figure 6.2 — and note that canola oil, just recently becoming widely available and made from rapeseed, has the least amount of saturated fat of anything on the market); then come oils high in monounsaturated plus polyunsaturated fatty acids (examples: sunflower, corn, and peanut oils). Oils high in saturated fatty acids (example: coconut oil) should be used as sparingly as possible.

The ideal cheese product is cheese curds — commonly known as cottage cheese — which have very little saturated fat. In most commercially made cottage cheese, the manufacturer has added some cream, which is why on its label it is called creamed cottage cheese. This does make it a little less of a low-fat food, but it is still one of the cheeses with the lowest fat content. Totally nonfat cottage cheese is also now commonly available in the major supermarkets. In commercially made buttermilk, manufacturers also often add a little cream, compromising its low-fatness slightly, but it too is still one of the lowest-fat dairy foods.

Which oil should you use and when? Here are some recommendations for general cooking:

1. Olive oil is excellent in salads, and is essential in many Italian recipes; it has its own distinctive flavor.

2. Corn oil is good for general cooking because it has little flavor of its own.

3. Peanut oil is good for stir-frying and other traditional Oriental dishes.

4. Canola oil is good for baked goods, salad dressings, sauces, and marinades.

Why the emphasis on types of fats and oils? Heart disease is less common among Mediterranean peoples than among northern Europeans or North Americans. Indeed, the incidence of cardiovascular disease and morbidity and mortality rates of Italian men and women are about half those found in the United States. Evidence now indicates that this is due to the higher relative consumption of monounsaturated fatty acids (i.e., olive oil) by Italian and Greek populations. Monounsaturated oils in the diet correlate with reduced levels of the LDL cholesterol which promotes heart disease, while keeping constant the HDL cholesterol that helps protect against heart disease. (Polyunsaturated oils tend to lower *both* LDL and HDL cholesterol). Recent evidence also suggests that monounsaturated oils are associated with lower blood pressures. So for daily eating you should shift, if you haven't already done so, toward a preponderance of monounsaturated oils. This doesn't mean you should begin dumping olive or canola oils on your food, since the *total amount* of fats and oils that you eat daily should be kept reasonably low.

Avoid processed and highly refined oils. Anything labeled simply "vegetable oil" is apt to be highly processed. Processed oils may be either hydrogenated or partially hydrogenated, which simply means that they have been converted from the original natural oil to a more saturated form of oil. Natural fatty acids exist in the chemical form known as cis, whereas in processed oils a substantial amount may have been converted to the trans form. The trans form appears to elevate serum cholesterol and LDL, and decrease HDL. "Trans" fats are even worse than saturated fats.

Italian olive oil is government regulated. The best quality, "extra virgin," is obtained by manual pressing of the olives between cold stone wheels. Excellent brands are Badic, Coltibuono, and Colavita. The best American olive oils are labeled "100 percent virgin," indicating that they are made from the first pressing of the olives, without additives, and that the oil is unrefined. These and other high-quality oils are not really expensive in proportion to the amount you use and they greatly enhance the flavor of the meal, so don't try to save money with lower-quality oils. Get the best! The terms "cold pressed" and "unrefined" as applied to American olive oils mean little, and are like the phony designation "natural" on many food products. Good American olive oils are Marsala and Sciabica.   Once opened, oils should be kept in the refrigerator to avoid oxidation.

Fish oil in the diet tends to protect against heart disease, due to its content of omega-3 fatty acids — the type found primarily in fish inhabiting deep cold waters: tuna, salmon, mackerel, herring, and sardines. The only fairly rich plant source of omega-3 fatty acids is the weedy herb purslane, sometimes added to salads. It's easy to grow if you have a garden, and was a favorite salad component in Biosphere 2, but it is generally not available in markets.

The first hint of the benefits of fish oil came from studies of Eskimos, who have a low incidence of arteriosclerosis despite eating a very high fat diet — but the fat they eat comes mostly from fish. In a ten-year-long study involving 6,000 middle-aged American men, a 40 percent lower mortality was found among those eating fish two to three times a week. In another study among 2,000 middle-aged men who had had one heart attack, those who were advised to eat two oil-rich fish meals per week displayed a 29 percent lower mortality rate over the succeeding two years. A few studies have suggested that fish in the diet may help lower blood pressure. The dietary supplement pills

MaxEPA and Promega are two good commercial sources of fish oils.

A note of caution: Large amounts of fish oils may decrease platelet aggregation and prolong bleeding time. Eskimos are known to bruise easily and to be liable to profuse nosebleeds. Aspirin also decreases platelet aggregation. High doses of fish oils should probably not be taken if one is taking aspirin; but two to three fish meals per week do not constitute a high dose. Four to six MaxEpa capsules per day would be a high dose. Also note, when buying canned fish packed in oil, the oil used is vegetable oil, not fish oil. The valuable fish oil is in the flesh of the fish itself.

Among vegetable oils, and for reasons that are not quite clear, monounsaturated fats seem somewhat superior to polyunsaturated fats in keeping arteriosclerosis to a minimum. Olive oil and canola have the highest percentages of monounsaturated fats (Fig 6.2).

Dietary Fat and Cancer

On the basis of population studies, it has been thought for some time that the total dietary fat level plays a significant role in suscepti-bility to cancers of the colon, breast, and stomach, and perhaps others. The message seems to be the more fat, the more cancer. Furthermore, these cancers have a low incidence in native Japanese, but high in the descendants of Japanese living in the United States who have adopted our diet. The genetic background is the same, but the cancer pattern follows the dietary pattern. And in Japan itself, as we have noted, the diet is changing, from the traditional diet of seafood, seaweed, vegeta-bles, rice, and beans to a more Western orientation. This is one of the less fortunate legacies of the American occupation after World War II. Between 1955 and 1988, fat consumption as a percentage of total calories tripled in Japan, and the major source of protein shifted from sea to land. There are hardly any fat Japanese in the over-60 age group — they still eat the traditional diet — but plenty of fat younger ones. There are now 706 outlets of an American fast-food hamburger chain in Japan, followed closely by outlets of an American fast-food fried-chicken chain.

Carbohydrates

About one fourth of the calories consumed by the average person today come from sugar, mainly hidden in processed foods and drinks.

Total average sugar intake has increased twenty-five fold during the past two hundred years. Sugar is the number one preservative used in today's processed foods. This is energy-rich but nutrient-poor consumption, exactly the reverse of healthy eating. Today we are eating foods with the highest calories and the lowest nutrients — foods that leave you hungry and, on a per-calorie basis, unnourished. By contrast, the foods of the Anti-Aging Plan give you the most satiation and nourishment in the most economical, calorie-rich form.

For many reasons, consumption of simple, refined sugars is bad for you. Refined sugars like sucrose (the one in your sugar bowl) tend to increase blood cholesterol. Cholesterol not only comes from the diet but also is synthesized by your liver, and refined sugar increases this internal synthesis; also, it lowers HDL. So if you think you have beaten the cholesterol problem by eating only lowfat foods, you may well be mistaken. Many of those lowfat foods are sweetened, and may for that reason increase internal cholesterol synthesis. A significant fact is that animals receiving sugar as part of their carbohydrate allowance have a shorter life span than those fed a complex carbohydrate, such as cornstarch, at the same calorie level.

One of the major modern theories of aging, the glycation theory, concerns excess sugar in the diet. Excess blood sugar slowly binds to proteins in our bodies, permanently altering their molecular structure. The proteins gradually turn yellow-brown, and their function is impaired. This process is called glycation.

A striking example of glycation concerns the proteins in the lens of the eye. Put the lens from a human eye into a concentrated solution of sugar and it gradually becomes cloudy and looks like a lens afflicted with cataract. People with diabetes, whose average blood sugar is way above normal, are five times as prone to develop cataract as other people. They also tend to show an increased susceptibility for developing arteriosclerosis.

The rate of glycation is determined by the concentration of sugar in the blood, and the length of time that it's elevated. Both of these factors are greatly increased when a high-sugar meal floods the blood with sugar and not enough insulin is present to distribute it to tissues at the normal rate.

Diabetics, whose insulin response is insufficient, show an enhanced rate of glycation of proteins. Diabetes is one of the diseases regarded as leading to accelerated aging.

And with age, normal people develop a response to sugar ingestion somewhat resembling diabetes.

Some proteins turn over quite rapidly in the body and are replenished, and for them glycation is not a serious problem.   Others are long-lived in the body, i.e., they do not turn over very rapidly.   Three such are crystallins in the lens of the eye, myelin in the sheaths around nerves, and the collagen of the connective tissue in skin, tendons, and the base membranes of the kidneys, as well as elsewhere throughout the body. Glycation of myelin may contribute to the nerve damage in diabetes and aging, of crystallin to the cataracts found in diabetes and in aging, and of collagen to arteriosclerosis and kidney damage.

We can to some extent reduce the progress of glycation by avoiding the eating habits that produce high glucose values. Simple carbohydrates — sugars like glucose, sucrose, and fructose —are the worst. Complex carbohydrates — especially those found in sweet potatoes, oats, apples, most kinds of beans, and brown rice — are much less prone to give elevated, protracted glucose levels. They comprised 75 to 80 percent of the calories eaten by the Biospherians, and contributed substantially to the remarkable 20 percent decline in Biospherian blood sugar levels reached by six months (Table 4.1).

An occasional high-fat and/or high-sugar dessert will not hurt you. If you feel you have a daily need for desserts, we predict that your adoption of the Anti-Aging Plan will at least decrease this need. And to satisfy whatever desire for sweets you do have, we suggest the dessert recipes in Part Two of this book (see Chapter 11).

Fiber

Fiber is very popular in lay nutritional literature today because the type and amount in the diet affects several physiological variables that in turn substantially influence health. Fiber influences the level of blood cholesterol, fecal bulk and colonic function, and blood sugar metabolism. Fortunately, fiber adds *no calories* to your diet.

Populations with a low average fiber intake show an increased frequency of heart disease, gallstones, diabetes, obesity, varicose veins, diverticulitis, hemorrhoids, and cancer of the bowel and, possibly, breast.

The term "fiber" itself makes one visualize long filaments of material resembling pieces of cornstalks or straw, or the insoluble cellulose strings in celery; but "fiber" also includes a number of gellike and mucilagenous materials like those found, for example, in cooked oat bran.

The term "fiber" refers to the portions of plants that mammals cannot digest, and which therefore cannot be absorbed from the human intestines. Fibers are the substances present in the cell walls that give plants their stucture and form. Dietary fiber, as the term is now used, is quite different from the older term, "crude fiber." Crude fiber values still appearing in many food tables are of little value. True dietary fiber may be four to five times as plentiful as "crude fiber."

Roughly speaking, there are two kinds of fiber: water soluble and insoluble. Water-soluble fiber helps lower blood cholesterol. Insoluble fibers help normalize bowel function and prevent bowel cancer and diverticulosis. In Finland, where the intake of both fiber and fat is high, the frequency of bowel cancer is low. The bad effects of fat in this one particular area of the body are canceled out by the high fiber intake.

Studies of populations from different countries have consistently shown an inverse correlation between fiber intake and death from heart disease. This is due to lowering of blood cholesterol by a diet high in soluble fibers. In one study, including 3.4 grams of the soluble fiber psyllium in the diet three times per day lowered blood cholesterol by 13 percent. The best-known brand name for psyllium is Metamucil. We recommend 5 to 10 grams of this or a generic equivalent per day. (Paradoxically, psyllium also improves bowel function, leading to bulkier softer stools, even though, on the whole, only insoluble fibers do this).

Soluble fibers probably exert their cholesterol-lowering effect by binding bile acids (which contain lots of cholesterol), which are then excreted rather than being reabsorbed in the intestines, by increasing breakdown of cholesterol in the liver, and probably through other mechanisms as well, such as altering fat absorption. Different soluble fibers may have quite different chemical structures. Soluble fibers are also associated with improved blood sugar regulation in diabetes. They slow down transit in the upper gut, a sort of viscous drag, and delay sugar absorption. It will be for future research to correlate structure and function of the different fibers. Oat bran has been considered among fiber-conscious eaters to be the richest source of soluble fiber, and to lower serum cholesterol. Another fiber paradox, however, is that rice bran, which is virtually devoid of soluble fiber, is superior as a cholesterol-lowering agent. The behavior of the soluble fiber psyllium on stool bulk and of the insoluble fiber from rice bran on cholesterol show that generalities don't always explain the influence of a specific type of fiber on physiology.

Wheat bran and wheat products, brown rice, and lentils are rich in insoluble fiber. Apples, bananas, citrus fruits, carrots, barley, and oats are rich in soluble fiber. Kidney beans, navy beans, green beans, and peas have lots of both types. But the categories of insoluble and soluble fibers are themselves divisible into quite different components. Only very broadly can it be said that *soluble* fibers in the diet influence blood cholesterol and hence heart disease, as well as blood sugar metabolism and hence the age-related tendency to diabetes. And only generally can it be said that *insoluble* fibers influence colon function and susceptibility to cancer of the large bowel.

Insoluble fibers exert their colon-protection effect(s) by increasing the bulk of the stool, increasing the amount of calcium in the large bowel, and decreasing the rate there of cell turnover. The stool-bulking effect of fiber may be more a matter of how much of the sugar pentose it contains, rather than its insolubility, which may be why the pentose-high soluble psyllium increases stool weight.

While Dr. Denis Burkett is credited in modern times with discovering the beneficial effects of high-fiber diets, he was not the first. Hippocrates wrote in 430 *B.C.* that "wholemeal bread clears out the gut and passes through as excrement." Hippocrates would not have liked white bread, or anything made from white flour. One cup of white flour has 3.0 grams of fiber, while the same amount of whole-wheat flour contains 14.5 grams. (Check the package labels to make sure what you are buying contains whole grains, of any type). Graham, who devised the first graham crackers, and Kellogg, the cereal man, also promoted dietary fiber, in the early 1900s.

Table 6.2 gives some examples of contents of soluble and insoluble fibers from selected foods.

Table 6.2
FIBER CONTENT OF SELECTED FOODS

	G sol. fiber	G insol. fiber
Apple (1)	0.9	2.1
Banana (1)	0.6	1.5
Fig (1)	3.7	2.9
Orange (1)	1.6	1.6
Prunes (3)	1.1	2.6
Broccoli (1/2 cup cooked)	0.9	1.1
Carrots (12 cup cooked)	1.1	1.2
Cauliflower (1/2 cup cooked)	0.5	1.1
Corn (1/2 cup cooked)	0.2	2.7
Green peas (1/2 cup cooked)	1.1	3.0
Potato, white (1)	1.8	2.0
Yam (1	3.0	2.8
Black-eyedpeas (1/2 cup cooked)	4.5	6.8
Kidney beans (1/2 cup cooked)	2.5	3.3
White beans (1/2 cup cooked)	1.5	3.5
Lentils (1/2 cup cooked)	0.5	2.5
Brown rice (1/2 cup cooked)	0.8	2.0
White rice (1/2 cup cooked)	0.0	0.2
Rolled oats (1/2 cup cooked)	0.8	1.6
Oat bran (1/2 cup cooked)	3.0	3.3
Wheat bran (1 Tblsp.)	0.5	3.0
White bread (1 slice)	0.2	0.2
Whole wheat bread (1 slice)	0.3	1.2

Nondigestible cellulose (high in bran, for example) increases fecal bulk and fluidity, but does not measurably affect blood cholesterol. Other kinds of fibers, the water-soluble, gel-forming pectins (in the white pith of citrus fruits and in bananas, carrots, and apples) and gums (found especially in legumes) lower both LDL and blood cholesterol primarily by interfering with fat absorption from the intestines, by slowing the rate of sugar absorption, and by binding with and increasing the secretion of bile acids.

Fiber also helps regulate appetite. It is filling but it adds *no calories* to the meal. In one study, the addition of 10 grams of guar gum fiber to meals twice daily decreased appetite by delaying gastric emptying time, decreased LDL fats in the blood, improved the glucose values, and led to significant weight loss in obese persons over a ten-week period.

The average daily intake of fiber in most Western diets is about 20 grams, much too low; in Third World countries, the intake is 60 grams.

If you are an average-size person, you should be consuming *at least* 40 grams of total fiber in your meals per day, but work up to it gradually to avoid temporary flatulence and bloating. For example, 1/2 cup cooked black beans, 2 slices whole-wheat bread, 1/4 cup rolled oats plus 1/4 cup oat bran, 1 medium sweet potato, 1 apple, 1 banana, 1/2 cup corn, 1/2 cup broccoli, 1 medium carrot, 1/2 cup green peas, or 1 tomato equals 40 grams of fiber. Most vegetarians consume considerably more than 40 grams per day. The Biospherian range was 45 to 60 grams per day. This played a role in their weight loss and contributed to marked improvement in both aging and biomarker health indices.

Nutrient-Richest Foods

The best foods are those which are the most nutrient rich, i.e., contain the highest amounts of essential nutrients *per calorie*. Broadly speaking, vegetables are clearly superior. Besides nutrient richness, they have the advantage of being low in fats, especially saturated fats, low in cholesterol, and high in fiber. A close second are legumes (beans of various types), and finally, complex carbohydrates.

Populations whose diets are rich in vegetables, fruits, and grains have significantly lower rates of cancer of the colon, breast, lung, mouth, esophagus, stomach, bladder, cervix, and pancreas. Remember, however, that limiting yourself entirely to vegetables would provide you with insufficient amounts of certain key substances, vitamin B12 for example. (We had to take B12 supplements in the Biosphere.) Other key substances you would lack in an all-vegetable diet would include niacin, folacin, riboflavin, magnesium, and the essential amino acids lysine and methionine. So you must combine vegetable foods with other types of food for complementarity.

Figure 6.3 lists recommended foods from different food categories, given on a "portion" basis (i.e., one portion equals one normal serving). The pluses in the table mean that the food is especially rich in the vitamin or mineral in that column, and the circles mean the food is moderately rich. Read this table. Let it guide your food selections for those meals where you are devising your own menus as a variation from the Anti-Aging Plan menus given in this book, in *Maximum Lifespan*, and in *The 120-Year Diet* (for complete bibliographical references to these other books see Appendix D).

The *Brassica* class of vegetables deserves special emphasis: kale, broccoli, collards, cauliflower, brussels sprouts, mustard greens and turnip greens in particular. Besides containing beta-carotene, vitamin C, and fiber in relatively high amounts, these are a good source of calcium, which is apt to be low if dairy products are only a small proportion of your diet. Note, however, that much of the calcium is contained in the leaves, rather than the stems of the plants. Thus, a serving of chopped frozen broccoli may contain more calcium than fresh broccoli, from which the leaves have often been plucked away. Some vegetables, like spinach, contain large amounts of oxalates, which limit calcium absorption from the gut. The above *Brassica* listed above do not contain oxalate, and their high calcium content is wholly absorbed.

Several studies have linked a reduction in cancer risk with consumption of large amounts of *Brassica* vegetables. This effect mainly obtains, however, only when they are eaten raw.

Supplementation

You want to get a full complement of the Recommended Daily Allowances (RDAs). You also want to be sure you are getting "safe and adequate" amounts of certain nutrients that have not yet made it into the "essential" category but that are still recognized as being potentially important. The official recommendations are those set forth by the National Academy of Sciences Nutrition Review Board.

However, in reviewing the data for establishing the RDAs and "safe and adequate" amounts, the Review Board, while employing six worthwhile criteria, has always neglected a seventh: What is the long-term effect of higher-than-RDA levels of nutrient essentials on disease resistance and longer life? They neglect this criterion because long-term data are not as yet conclusive. But research in this direction has become much more respectable than it once was, and beneficial effects

Range of RDA's per portion / Food	Portion Wt. (gms)	Cals.	vit. A	vit. C	vit. D	vit. E	vit. K	Thia-mins	Ribo-flavin	Niacin	B-6	Panto-thenic acid	B-12	Fola-cin
Banana	150	127									+			
Cantaloupe	200	60	+	+										
Papaya	100	39	•	+										
Millet	100	327						•	•		+			
Rice – brown	100	356									•	•		
Rice – wild	100	353						•	•	•		•		
Wheat germ	10	40				+	•							
Whole wheat pasta	80	266						•						
Kombu	8	19			•						•		•	
Nori	8	20	•		•						•		•	
Wakami	8	20			•					•			•	
Brewer's yeast	10	56						+	•	•		•		
Beef (lean)	100	143				•				•			+	+
Chicken (dark)	100	130											+	+
Chicken (light)	100	117											+	+
Liver	100	140	+			+	+	+		•	+		+	+
Pork (lean)	100	165									•		+	+
Veal	100	156				•				•			+	+
Cod	100	78								+	+		+	+
Mackerel	100	191									+		+	+
Oysters	50	33				•				+	+			
Salmon	100	217											+	+
Sardines, fresh	50	78	•								+		+	
Sardines, canned	100	200		+										
Squid	100	84					+						+	+
Tuna	100	127				•					+		+	+
Skim milk	1 cup 244	85		+									+	
Buttermilk	244	100		+									+	
Yogurt	244	156		+		•							+	
Ricotta cheese (part skim)	1/2 cup 124	174		+									+	

Figure 6.3 Top quality food according to nutrient density per portion (+ = very high, • = high).

are being sorted out.

Vitamin C is a good example. The current RDA is 60 mg per day. That's quite adequate to prevent scurvy, but it does not address the question of whether animals or humans on larger doses over the whole course of their lives might have fewer diseases or live longer.

The RDAs may thus be looked upon as in most cases adequate but in some cases merely minimum values. This lack of pertinent scientific data does not justify indiscriminate megadosing of vitamins, minerals, or other supplements. In some cases, however, we are now able to make new judgments based on information in the medical and biological literature. We shall recommend taking RDA amounts of most essential and several other nutrients, and substantially increased amounts of a few.

Vitamins and Minerals That We Recommend Supplementing Beyond Recommended Daily Allowance Levels

Beta-carotene

Beta-carotene, which occurs naturally in certain foods, is the strongest available antioxidant for "singlet oxygen," a very damaging and mutagenic (cancer-causing) form of free radical. So-called free radicals are actively damaging side products of metabolism, which may be instrumantal in aging, and are certainly instrumental in a number of diseases. Free radicals are also present in cigarette smoke and air pollutants in industrial cities. And there are a number of different kinds. A portion of ingested beta-carotene is converted in the body into vitamin A, but only upon demand. Too much vitamin A is toxic, but beta-carotene by itself is virtually nontoxic. The unconverted beta-carotene remains stored in the tissues, where it functions as an antioxidant. Taking beta-carotene thus covers both your vitamin A needs and has additional potential value. It was found in The Physicians Health Study that those taking beta-carotene experienced only half as many vascular events (heart attacks, strokes) as controls.

We recommend taking 25,000 IUs (international units) per day. Very high doses (much higher than what we are recommending here) have the side effect of turning the skin slightly yellow-orange, but even this is harmless and will disappear if the large amount is discontinued.

The Biospherian diet was extremely high in beta-carotene, and we did turn slightly orange during the course of the experiment.

Vitamin E

Free radicals can form a self-generating, self-damaging chain reaction in the body. Vitamin E is the only fat-soluble antioxidant normally present in human blood that breaks this chain. It has not been shown to influence maximum life span, but it substantially retards buildup of the yellow-brown so-called age pigment that accumulates with time in the brain, heart, liver, and testes. Also, it partially protects animals from poisoning by chemical agents such as mercury, lead, carbon tetra-chloride, and possibly ozone, nitrogen dioxide, and paraquat.

Larger-than-RDA amounts of vitamin E increases the immune response in humans; and in animal experiments, for example, large amounts of vitamin E in the diet have given a fourfold increase in survival from pneumonia.

About 300 IUs per day seems optimal for immunologic stimulation in humans. It comes in a number of forms. We recommend the vitamin E succinate or vitamin E acetate forms.

Vitamin C

Of all supplementary agents, vitamin C has been the most controversial, stemming in part from Dr. Linus Pauling's thesis that it helps prevent cancer. Pauling himself takes 15 grams per day, over two hundred times the RDA amount of 60 milligrams. His own experimental work dealing with the effect of oral vitamin C on development of spontaneous cancer in mice seems to support his thesis. Beyond that, there is insufficient experimental laboratory work on the question, partly because most animals make their own vitamin C in their bodies. It's only humans, other primates, and a few other species that don't. So we have no good, inexpensive mammalian model for extended experimental studies.

Do large doses of vitamin C influence cancer susceptibility? They do reduce the number of rats developing colon cancer in response to a chemical carcinogen. And vitamin C reduces the incidence of abnormalities in the DNA (the genetic material, abnormalities of which are often associated with later cancer development) of human workers exposed to coal tar products.

The National Research Council does now (finally) recommend eating plenty of vitamin C-containing foods, which in fact would result in more than the RDA amount in the diet, although they are not so bold as to flat-out increase the time-honored RDA recommendation. It is interesting that the human RDA has been set by the Food and Nutrition Board to about 60 mg, based on the amount needed to prevent scurvy in young men, whereas the Committee on Animal Nutrition recommends over ten times that amount for monkeys, based on the amounts required for optimal growth rate, wound healing rates, and resistance to infection. Humans and monkeys are close enough on the animal scale that their vitamin C needs should be similiar.

Besides being required for the formation of connective tissue (vitamin C's basic function), vitamin C stimulates the immune system and can act as a free radical scavenger. These constitute its so-called pharmacological properties — properties above and beyond its basic physiological function. In doses of 500 to 1000 mg daily, vitamin C has been shown in both human and animal experiments to decrease blood cholesterol.

Some evidence suggests that more-than-RDA amounts of vitamin C and beta-carotene may help prevent cataracts (which afflict 18 percent of Americans over age 65), and possibly macular degeneration in the eye (afflicting 28 percent of people over age 75, and the commonest cause of blindness in older Americans). The retina of the eye has a twenty times higher concentration of vitamin C than the blood, and presumably this serves some purpose. The sun's ultraviolet rays oxidize the lens's protein, leading eventually to cataracts. Free radical scavengers like vitamin C may help prevent this.

We recommend taking about 0.5 grams (500 mg) of vitamin C per day. If you do this, it is important to do it every day rather than on a hit or miss basis. Excess vitamin C is excreted rapidly, and once the excretory machinery is revved up, it keeps going. If you take a large amount for two or three days, and then forget, on the fourth day you may be in deficit. Alternating excess and deficit is not what you want.

Selenium

Selenium is a component of one of the body's major natural antioxidant (free radical scavenging) enzymes (glutathione peroxidase). While the evidence for its having a life span prolonging effect is marginal, the evidence that fairly high levels of selenium in a person's food intake exerts an anti-cancer effect is quite substantial. High selenium intake correlates with lower incidence of breast cancer. In the United States, when the selenium levels in the blood of people from different regions is compared with the overall cancer death rates in those regions, the rates are lower where the selenium in the soil and crops is higher. And in general, people developing cancer had low blood selenium levels well before the onset of the cancer. Animal data supports these human studies. Finally, selenium deficiency is associated with an excessive risk of heart attack.

We recommend supplementation with 100 micrograms of selenium per day, in the organic form. Studies from China do indicate that 800 micrograms per day may have toxic effects. You should stay well below that level, and since the amount in your food may vary, it is best not to exceed our 100 micrograms of extra supplementation. The product you are buying should say "organically bound" on the label. If it says "added to" or "fortified," it is the least desirable brand to buy.

Additional Vitamins and Minerals

There is some evidence, but less strong than for those discussed above, that supplementation with a few other vitamins and minerals beyond the RDA recommendations might have additional health benefits. These other vitamins and minerals are magnesium, chromium, niacin, bioflavinoids, and vitamin B6. Note, however, that for these vitamins and minerals early evidence has not been followed up by more rigorous studies. One can only make a presumptive judgment and be careful not to overdo the amount taken.

Magnesium intake in the United States has been declining since 1900 in the face of increases in intake of substances that augment the need for it, such as vitamin D in fortified milk and phosphorus in soft drinks. Long-term inadequacy of magnesium appears associated with heart disease. It is probably the ratio of magnesium to calcium that exerts this effect. Supplementation with 0.5 to 1 gram of magnesium per day would seem potentially beneficial.

The trace element chromium is responsible for the biologic activity of the so-called glucose tolerance factor, or GTF, deficiency of which may play a role in late-onset diabetes. Chromium is usually deficient in the average American diet. In one study, up to 90 percent of individuals were found to be consuming less than the minimum suggested "safe and adequate" amounts. Chromium is present in high amounts in brewer's yeast. Chromium is a required co-factor for the action of insulin, which influences especially carbohydrate but also protein and fat metabolism. It increases lean body mass (i.e., lowers the percentage of body fat), lowers blood glucose, and decreases glycated hemoglobin. The picolinate form is best. We recommend supplementation in the amount of 200 micrograms per day.

Large doses of niacin increase the level of HDL in the blood by as much as 30 percent, and decrease the cholesterol/HDL ratio by an average of 25 percent. These changes would correspond to a substantial decrease in susceptibility to heart disease. The doses required, however, vary from 250 mg to 1 gram per day, which in many persons leads to severe upper body flushing, itching, and gastrointestinal symptoms. We do not recommend niacin supplementation at this time, unless by your doctor's decision.

One can make an arguable case for more than RDA supplementation with a few other materials, pantothenic acid and vitamin B6 for example. But the evidence is marginal as to long-term benefits, and you need not supplement your diet further, assuming you are eating a balanced mixture of wholesome foods. There is, however, no objection to a daily multivitamin-mineral supplementation in not greater than RDA amounts, if you are so inclined.

Which Brand?

In this regard, we are often asked which company to buy from. In judging this, you should inspect the label on the bottle. The label is covered by government regulations, whereas accompanying promotional literature is much less regulated. If you have a choice, always buy products whose labels show an expiration date. This guarantees full potency up to that date. Thompson, Bronson, and Twin Labs all produce multivitamin/multimineral capsules or tablets containing approximately 100 percent of the RDA of these essential nutrients. Beta-carotene, vitamin E, vitamin C, and chromium picolinate can be taken separately.

Other Supplements

A number of other drugs and medicaments are on the market, with various claims as to their efficacy in retarding aging or having other

health benefits: centrofenoxine, DMAE, L-dopa, centrofenoxine, pirace-
tum, choline, hydergine, vasopressin, deprenyl, and various antioxidants. While one can make a theoretical case for many of these, certainly the essential evidence must come from long-term studies in animals, both with regard to population survival curves and incidence of
the diseases of aging. These have either not been done or produced
evidence that is at best marginal.

It is interesting to note, however, that a number of respected phar-
maceutical and newly formed "venture capital" firms (Odyssey
Therapeutics, for example) are moving actively into the search for, and
— what is most important — reliable testing of, anti-aging drugs. This
is a new phenomenon and bodes well.

We do recommend Coenzymne Q10 as a supplement. CoQ10, as it
is called, is an essential part of the membranes of the energy factories
of the cell, and may also have some antioxidant functions. In the initial
aging study with CoQ10, weekly injections of 17-month-old mice led to
a substantial increase in their survival compared to noninjected controls.[6] In studies by Dr. Steve Harris at UCLA, inclusion of CoQ10 in
the diet led to some extension of the average life spans of mice.
Furthermore, older mice with CoQ10 in their diet appeared substantially younger than controls. More work needs to be done, and the jury
is still out, but since CoQ10 is a nontoxic normal constituent of the
body, we recommend the inclusion of 20 mg per day as dietary supplementation.

A major study completed several years ago at Harvard Medical
School indicated that taking one aspirin every other day will substantially reduce the chance of a heart attack. Indeed, after four years the
incidence of first-time heart attacks was slashed by 44 percent. Aspirin
helps delay clot formation, and most heart attacks stem from the formation of a clot upon the rough lining of an arteriosclerotic heart vessel. Aspirin has no effect upon the genesis of arteriosclerosis itself.
Reducing the risk of getting arteriosclerosis is more important in the
long run than preventing a clot. The Anti-Aging Plan will substantially
reduce that risk. Also, aspirin has some serious side effects, and should

[6] E. G. Bliznakoff, *Biomedical and Clinical Aspects of Coenzyme Q.*vol.3
(Elsevier/Amsterdam, 1981), p.311.

not be taken if you have high blood pressure, ulcers, any kind of bleeding disorder, liver disease, kidney disease, or gout. In any case, be sure to obtain your doctor's approval before taking aspirin on a daily basis.

Alcoholic Beverages

Alcohol is hardly a nutrient-rich food, in fact quite the opposite, but a glass of good beer, wine, scotch, or whatever you prefer, need not upset your program. If you are losing weight a bit too rapidly on a nutrient-rich diet of, say, 1800 calories per day, but fulfilling all your RDA requirements, you might choose to add 100 to 200 calories from alcoholic beverages. This would be one to two drinks per day. We do not encourage this, but it is much healthier than adding sugar, for example, since a modest amount of alcohol in this diet does correlate with a somewhat lower incidence of heart disease. In a word, alcohol in small amounts is the least injurious material in the empty-calorie category.

Be aware that a number of domestic beers and wines contain chemical additives — up to fifty-two chemical ingredients are permitted in domestic beers, and over sixty-two in wines. Most of these, like citric acid and corn syrup used as flavoring agents, are harmless. Others, like sodium metabisulfite, can cause allergic reactions. Some of the "light" beers are the worst offenders. If you like beer, drink German beer. A German law enacted four hundred years ago prohibits adding anything to the hops, barley, and malt that go into the making of beer. A similar law against additives holds for wines in France.

Restaurants and Eating Away from Home

You can eat quite delicious meals away from home without giving up the Anti-Aging Plan. Here is how: First, if you are eating the diet with caloric limitation added for lifespan extension, *don't think about the total number of calories* you are eating when you dine out. Don't carry a calorie book or a foodscale along with you. There is simply no need for this kind of constant exact monitoring of intake. By sheer habit you will be able to estimate your intake with reasonable accuracy, and besides, eating away from home often coincides with occasions when food is a special event — holiday meals, or meals in fine restaurants — and precise counting of calories (not to mention the amused stares of your fellow diners) would spoil the event.

However, you can and should still focus on the *quality* of your menu selections. If you are really eating the Anti-Aging Plan's nutrient -rich food combinations daily, then you will have discovered the superior and satisfying tates of these foods. Nutrient rich foods can be great treats, and will be more and more available as many of the leading chefs of the world concentrate (as they are beginning to do) on low-calorie, low-fat gourmet cuisine. You can find such food in a number of restaurants today: Panache's in Los Angeles, for example, or the so-called Spa cuisine at the Four Seasons in New York. In any case, the key to eating out is: Focus not on calorie count but rather on *calorie quality*; and then, within reason, eat as much as you like. This assumes, of course, you are eating dinner out once or twice a week, not every night.

At the restaurant select steamed, broiled, roasted, or poached menu items, and avoid sauteed, fried, braised, creamed, or escalloped items. Some restaurants, especially hotel restaurants, offer low-calorie, low-fat meals, often of very good quality. These are usually indicated on the menu. Even the fast food chains now offer low-fat items. Some of the hamburger chains provide burgers made with lean beef, and have salad bars. Some of the fried chicken chains offer skinless fried chicken, which is lower in fat. Many of the soft-ice-cream chains now offer low-fat ice cream, low-fat frozen yogurt, and even nonfat frozen desserts.

Two important tips:
1. Most restaurants bring bread to the table as soon as you sit down. Don't fill up on bread and butter while waiting for the first course. Wait until your entree comes before having a serving of bread.
2. A major item of restaurant fare is the potato. A medium-size potato is quite nutritious by itself, containing lots of potassium, vitamin C, vitamin B6, and fiber and trace minerals, all for just 150 calories and with no fat at all. But butter, sour cream, cheese (usually in stuffed restaurant potatoes), or french frying turn the potato into a high-calorie, high-fat artery clogger. For restaurant dining, select a baked potato and top it with a few items from the salad bar (tomato, mushroom, onion, sprouts) and a little yogurt, and you will have a nutient-rich combination.

Airline Meals

If you fly a lot, you should be aware that most airlines, including many international carriers, offer quite an array of special meals. This is a rather well-kept secret because the meals require special handling. But they are available to help you stay on your diet while flying, and they are often tastier than the primary airline fare. You must, however, inform the airline of what you want twenty-four hours in advance.

The airline meal types can be divided into religious (kosher, Hindu, Muslim), medical (low-sugar, low-cholesterol, low-calorie, low-fat, low-sodium), and others (fruit plate, hot or cold seafood, strict vegetarian, and ovo/lacto vegetarian). Here are some specialty airline meals typically offered, plus the names they go by on the airline roster: "low-fat" dinner (baked chicken, mixed vegetables, broiled tomato, fruit salad); vegetarian dinner (vegetarian stuffed pepper, salad, broth, and bread); cold seafood plate (seafood salad, shrimp, cocktail sauce, tomatoes, fresh fruit, dessert). Each time you fly try a different one, and find what you like.

Chapter 7

Seven Simple Steps

In this chapter we give you step by step instructions on how to begin and continue the health-promoting, life-extending Anti-Aging Plan. You will find the meal plan easy, pleasurable, and nutritionally sound. Details and explanations are given elsewhere in the book. Here in a few words is what you do.

Step 1

Buy a good scale and weigh yourself once a week, on the same day each week, at the same time in the morning before breakfast. Decide whether you are going (a) for gradual weight loss and health promotion only, eating as much as you want of the foods in the plan; or (b) for weight loss, health promotion, and also life span extension by eating the Anti-Aging Plan with caloric limitation. If you choose the added benefit of life span extension, you must now gauge your individual set-point, according to principles given in Chapter 5. You may choose anywhere from a 10 percent to a 20 percent loss of your set-point body weight. The Anti-Aging Plan sets this limit of a 20 percent reduction of your set-point body weight for overall well-being and normal daily living in society; any greater reduction than this should be avoided. You may expect to lose weight fairly rapidly during the first four weeks, but after that your rate of weight loss should be slow. Remember: *Very slow and steady weight loss* is the way to reap life span extension from the Anti-Aging Plan practiced with caloric limitation.

Step 2

Consult a doctor whom you trust and who is receptive at the very least to the health benefits of the Anti-Aging Plan without caloric limitation. And if you are choosing to add caloric limitation for life span extension, definitely tell your doctor this. Whether or not he or she agrees with the plan's potential for life span extension, he or she must advise you on your eligibility to adopt a meal plan of caloric limitation, based on the status of your health. Note: If you are pregnant or a nursing mother, you definitely should not adopt the Anti-Aging Plan with caloric limitation during this time.

Have a general checkup. This should include your blood pressure, pulse, cholesterol, HDL, fasting blood sugar, tests for autoantibodies, and a white blood cell count. Ask your doctor to tell you the results. Record these for your own future reference. Run these tests again four to six months after you have started the diet, and at least once a year thereafter. The other biomarkers and health indicators given in Chapter 4 are optional, but get them if you can.

If you are consistently carrying out the Anti-Aging Plan's meal plan (an *occasional* splurge on a rich or nonnutrient-rich food is all right), you should notice within two to six months not only weight loss, but also lowered blood pressure, lowered pulse rate, and a substantially lowered blood cholesterol. Fasting blood sugar will be somewhat decreased, autoantibody tests negative, and white blood cell count near the low side of normal or actually less than normal. If these changes have occurred, you are doing well. Already, you have undergone a veritable makeover. Keep it up.

Step 3

To start your changeover to the Anti-Aging Plan's nutrient-rich meal plan, you may choose between the two methods detailed in Chapter 5. If you want to rev your motor before your changeover to a full-time meal plan, we suggest Method 1, Rapid Reorientation: For four weeks adhere rigorously to the foods, menus and food combinations given in this book (See Chapters 10 and 11). You will experience a quite stimulating reorientation of your food habits, and you will also achieve considerable weight loss. As you progress through these four weeks of Rapid Reorientation, you'll be referring increasingly to the sample menus in Appendix C.

If you do not choose to rev your engine before starting your changeover, then we recommend Method 2, Gradual Reorientation. Here is how: Cook once a week, as detailed in Chapter 5, eight meals of which seven can be frozen, using the recipes in Chapter 10. We recommend this Quantity-Cook-and-Freeze option because it will guarantee you a smooth, steady, secure, and successful transition to the meal plan full-time. The nutrient-rich meals will be at your fingertips, ready to eat, which is a big advantage when you are doing a makeover of your personal daily meal plan.

In your very first week, start gradually. Select one afternoon of that week. On that afternoon — say, Saturday — prepare eight and freeze seven separate portions of your selected nutrient-rich meal. On the following Monday, which will be the beginning of your first week, eat one of these portions for either lunch or dinner, and for the other meals of that particular day eat wholesome foods.

The rest of that first week, eat as you are accustomed to doing. There is no big hurry.

The second Saturday prepare eight and freeze seven portions of another nutrient-rich meal from Chapter 10. On the following Monday and Tuesday eat a portion of your two prepared meals for either lunch or dinner, and wholesome foods the rest of those days.

The following Saturday prepare a third meal, and add Wednesday to your Anti-Aging Plan days.

By the seventh week (1) you will be eating nutrient-rich meals full-time, seven days a week, and (2) you will have a freezerful of entrees that will never be depleted, as long as you keep replenishing it on your one cooking day per week.

For the rest of the day before and after your one-a-day nutrient-rich meal, simply eat wholesomely and sensibly. The Free-Choice Recipes in Chapter 11 are very good choices for wholesome, sensible gourmet eating. For your daily meal plan, follow the general principles detailed in Chapter 6. Eat the low-calorie Miracle Soup (page 190) between meals if you feel hungry or need a snack. Your other meal choices should be low in fat, with a shift toward quality fats (Chapter 6 will tell you what we mean by "quality fats"). Find restaurants in your city that offer this kind of food on a gourmet basis. Nowadays, even the inexpensive fast-food chains offer lean dishes and sumptuous salad bars. If you travel a lot, ask the airlines for special meals.

One of the healthiest of all foods is brewer's yeast. If you like its nutty taste, eat two tablespoonfuls per day, sprinkled on your morning cereal, for example, or stirred into a citrus juice.

Step 4

As you become more familiar with the diet, you may also wish to devise your own 50% RDA nutrient-rich meals. This can be done manually by using good nutrient tables (see references in Appendix D), or quite easily, if you have a computer, by means of available nutrition software that we detail in Appendix B.

Too much caffeine is not beneficial, but coffee or tea with milk are okay in moderation. No sugar or cream, however!

By this time, you will actually be on the Anti-Aging nutrient-rich meal plan full-time. Assuming that you are using the One-A-Day Meal Method (implemented most easily by the Quantity-Cook-and-Freeze Option), your stomach should be satisfied and happy.

Avoid sugar and other simple carbohydrates, including honey, as much as possible. Nonfat dairy products are okay but be moderate with other dairy products. To have the largest quantity of food that gives you the maximum satiation is simply to eat plant foods mainly, rather than foods having an animal source. Eat animal-derived foods as *accompanying items*, but base your meal on plant-originated foods — grains, beans, rice, pasta, breads, starchy vegetables, green vegetables, fruits.

Keep weighing yourself once a week. Your goal is gradual loss of weight on a high-quality, nutrient-rich diet. Remember: the guiding principle in extending life span is total calorie intake rather than where the calories come from, but on this lower calorie intake your food *must* be nutrient-packed, nutrient-rich. You must never be nutrient-deficient, nutrient-poor. The nutrient-packed calorie that you eat will give you a sense of satisfaction and well-being.

You'll live longer, you'll need less sleep, you'll have a sharper mind, you'll feel better, you'll get fewer colds, flus, and be generally less susceptible to other diseases.

If you like creating recipes, create your own new One-A-Day Meals by computer along the principles given in Appendix B.

Step 5

With your doctor's approval, begin a program of moderate exercise, more or less equivalent to fifteen miles of jogging per week. If you are not a lover of exercise, the easiest way to do this is to take a brisk thirty-minute walk three times per week. Walking is a comfortable form of exercise even for very overweight people. Choose a place to walk that is safe and without too many stoplight crosswalks, which would force you to stop and wait and interrupt the pleasant swing and rhythm of your walking. If you change the routes you take in your walks, they will not get boring.

Step 6

For supplementation, take one multivitamin/mineral tablet per day that gives you approximately 50 percent of the RDAs and "safe and adequate" amounts of the essential vitamin and mineral nutrients. In addition, take 0.5 gram of vitamin C, 300 to 400 units of vitamin E, 100 micrograms of selenium, 25,000 units of beta-carotene. Also, 0.5 to 1 grams of magnesium per day, 0.1 mg of chromium in the organic form per day, and 20 mg of CoQ10 per day are safe, but optional, since the evidence about their benefits is less conclusive.

Step 7

As a final step: Make plans for what you want to do with your better body and your longer, healthier, more vigorous life.

BOOK TWO

RECIPES

Chapter 8

Your Nutrient-Rich Kitchen: Supplies and Basic Equipment

In this chapter we will tell you how to set up your kitchen, what equipment and basic supplies you need for a full go at the Anti-Aging Plan. We don't expect you to rush forth and buy all these items before you cook your first meal. These are merely the items you will begin to accumulate as you progress with the program.

Remember that the basic plan is to cook eight portions of one nutritionally rich dish once per week, and freeze seven of them. The first two weeks we suggest that you cook at least twice, in quanitity. You thereby gradually accumulate a number of high-quality frozen dishes. These meals are generally one-dish recipes designed with the help of a computer to fulfill at least 60 percent of your daily requirements for vitamins, minerals, and amino acids, while limiting the percentage of calories from fat to below 20 percent. Once you have properly equipped your kitchen, quantity cooking is not much more time-consuming than regular cooking.

Ingredients

The particular ingredients in the One-A-Day Megameals and in the Free-Choice Recipes are essential both for superb flavor and for their remarkable nutritional values. Remember that the anti-aging recipes add nutritional completeness to the flavors of each dish; nutritional density is a vital element in the Anti-Aging Plan. Once you are familiar with the preparation of these ingredients, you will probably want to add them to many of your own recipes. For rural readers, we have referenced several mail-order companies in Appendix A to help you locate these essential foods.

In the Megameals we have included modified versions of classic American and European traditional meals, as well as modified versions of traditional meals from other countries.

What amazed us as we developed the Megameals was the similarity in food ingredients from country to country. While each ethnic cuisine may have its own seasonings, methods of cutting and preparing foods, still there are really only a finite number of foods available on the earth. Hence, nutritionally speaking, a Spanish Paella is very similar to an Indonesian Pullao, or a Turkish/Persian Pilaf. And a Mexican Burrito is very similar to Chinese Mu Shu vegetable (or chicken) or a French chicken-stuffed Crêpe.

The Anti-Aging kitchen is like any other kitchen in the sense that it is full of staples; it is new and improved in the sense that it is the sum total of all kitchens from all over the world! It is a well-stocked yet economical pantry. Following are some checklists for accumulating and organizing what you need.

The Pantry

•Alphabetize your spices.
•Hang your favorite pots and pans from a pegboard attached to the kitchen wall.
•Hang small, frequently used kitchen tools from the same board.

A well-organized pantry not only makes cooking easier, *it also makes meal-planning much easier.* If foods are intelligently arranged and labeled in big letters (remember, many grains look alike in a glass canister), you can stand before your cupboard shelves, breezily scan them, and get fresh cooking ideas. This goes for equipment organization, too.

•Buy one-quart canning jars and stick on large-lettered labels for your grains, pastas, and legumes (beans). In larger containers store pastas, rice, bran, and flour. Store seaweeds, dried chilies, and dried mushrooms in sealed containers to discourage insects.

Foodstuffs to Keep on Hand

Grains and Cereals

Brown rice
Wild rice
Barley
Buckwheat
Bulgur
Couscous
Millet
Rolled oats
Wheat bran

Flour and Pasta

Whole-wheat flour
Oat flour
Whole-wheat pastry flour
Cornmeal
Whole-wheat pasta (spaghetti, macaroni, lasagne, shells)
Brown rice pasta
Soba noodles

Legumes

Black beans
Black-eyed peas
Garbanzo beans
Kidney beans
Lentils
Lima beans
White beans
Pinto beans
Soybeans

Nuts and Seeds

Almonds
Filberts (hazelnuts)
Walnuts
Pumpkin seeds
Sesame seeds
Sunflower seeds
Peanut butter
Sesame butter (tahini)

Seaweeds

Kombu
Nori
Arame

Oils

Canola oil spray
Olive oil spray
Olive oil
Sesame oil
Walnut oil

Dried Fruits

White figs
Papaya
Raisins
Currants

Dry Staples

Nonfat dry milk
Tapioca
Dried vege broth
Dried chicken broth

Brewer's yeast
Thickeners (arrowroot, cornstarch)
Baking powder
Baking soda
Shiitake mushrooms
Chinese dried mushrooms
Cream of tartar

Canned Staples

Evaporated skim milk
Tomato products
Green chilies and salsa
Sardines (packed in water)
Tuna (packed in water)
Chestnuts
Legumes
Water chestnuts
Artichoke hearts

Condiments and Flavorings

Vinegars (balsamic, raspberry,
 rice wine, cider, tarragon)
Dijon mustard
Capers
Hot sauce
Low-sodium soy sauce
Lemon, lime juice
Sake
Cooking wine
Vanilla

Frozen foods

Corn
Peas
Juices (orange, pineapple, apple)

Chopped spinach

Herbs

Basil
Bay leaves
Chives
Cilantro
Dill
Dried horseradish
Garlic powder
Marjoram
Dried mustard
Onion powder
Oregano
Rosemary
Sage
Tarragon
Thyme

Spices

Allspice
Black mustard seed
Cardamom
Cloves
Chili powder
Cinnamon
Coriander
Cumin
Fennel seed
Ginger
Nutmeg
Paprika
Pepper (black, white, cayenne)
Red pepper flakes
Saffron
Turmeric

Basic Equipment

Small Appliances: An electric blender, a food processor, and a smaller electric mini-chopper are so useful in nutrient-rich cooking that we would almost call them essential. If you do not have them, of course you can still do any of our megarecipes, but these machines are true time and labor savers.

Cookware: Because the Quantity-Cook-And-Freeze Option is such a time saver, invest in some large cookware for quantity meal preparation. It's worth it. The following is merely a suggestion: two-and four-quart saucepans; small, medium and large nonstick skillets; a large wok, as well as a large stockpot (8 quarts) for soups and pasta; two loaf pans (pyrex is fairly easy to clean); two 8" x 8" baking dishes, one or two 13" x 8" baking dishes; two large pie or quiche dishes, a nonstick cookie sheet; a broiler pan, an angel food nonstick cake pan. Bowls in a variety of sizes, and measuring cups.

Gadgets: Garlic press, ginger grater, cheese grater, salad spinner, colander/strainer, strong wire-mesh strainer for squeezing juice from pulp, kitchen timer, bulb baster, vegetable brush, wooden spoons (for cooking on nonstick surfaces), kitchen shears, wire whisk, good knives, spatulas, and an assortment of serving utensils. Include a wood cutting board for poultry along with your vegetable cutting board.

Cookbook holder: Lucite cookbook holders are practical and commercially available. Buy one. Then find a spot at eye level on your kitchen wall, where you can rest it.

Weighing Scale: Once familiar with Anti-Aging Plan cooking, you will rarely need to use a scale. Initially, however, we recommend that you do weigh some foods. We weigh brans, seaweeds, meats, and fish (if prepackaged). Most ingredients in these recipes are in standard measurements and won't need weighing.

Chapter 9

Tips, Tricks, Techniques, and Shortcuts

In this chapter we have gathered together all of our modern, sometimes revolutionary, and always tried-and-tested information on nutrient-rich food preparation. We open the chapter with nine foods that easily boost every recipe they are added to. We'll explain nurtritionally what each food supports you with as well as how to select, store, and prepare it. For maximum information retrieval, we have organized our information by subject, alphabetically.

This chapter is divided into three sections: **Nutrient Superchargers, Cooking Tips**, and **Freezing Tips** (for our Quantity-Cook-And-Freeze Option). We suggest that you read this section all the way through. It will give you ideas on how to translate many traditional cooking methods into an anti-aging cuisine. Please also refer to the Anti-Aging Glossary of Foods, for additional information about nutrient-rich food preparation.

NUTRIENT SUPER-CHARGERS

Bran Flakes; Oat and Wheat Bran

Bran flakes are the skin or husks of the grain kernel. They add a substantial amount of fiber to your diet. Fiber is the part of the plant that is not digested in the small intestine. It passes on to the large intestine (colon), where it promotes fecal bulk and acts as a natural laxative. Wheat bran is an insoluble fiber, while oat bran contains both insoluble and soluble fiber. Insoluble fiber absorbs water and passes through the digestive system unchanged. Its main dietary bonus is as a natural laxative and in its potential importance in preventing cancer of the colon. Soluble fibers have been found to reduce both cholesterol and blood sugar levels. Blood cholesterol levels and fasting blood sugar levels dropped significantly for all eight Biospheriens.

One heaping tablespoon of bran will supply 10 percent of your daily nutritional requirements for fiber. We recommend that you use oat bran whenever possible and wheat bran flakes as an alternative. Simply add it to whatever you are preparing. Sprinkle it over cereal, into a soup or salad, or add a few tablespoons to beans and casseroles while cooking. Bran flakes are neutral and will not alter the taste of your recipe.

If you have a hard time finding oat bran, it is available through the mail-order references in Appendix A. And don't worry. Soluble fiber is readily available in the plant kingdom in the form of apples, carrots, broccoli, and beans, to name only a few. Wheat bran is an alternative and is commercially available in most supermarkets. Bran flakes should be stored in an airtight container and will keep indefinitely.

Kombu

Kombu is a seaweed liberally used in Japanese preparation of soups. A small 2-gram piece, a 3" x 1" strip boasts 27 percent of your RDA for vitamin D (a vitamin important in the absorption of calcium and difficult to get in unfortified foods) and 20 percent of your daily needs for calcium.

Kombu comes in long strips that are dried and sold in 1-and 2-ounce packages in health food stores and in the Asian section of your supermarket. If you can't find it, check Appendix A. We list a mail order company that does sell kombu.

If used in stews or soups, kombu should be cut with kitchen shears while still dry and added in the first stages of cooking your soup. For stir-frys or casseroles, cover the strips completely with water and soak them for 10 or 15 minutes. Kombu will swell to twice its original size, and can easily be minced once softened. Don't be put off by the texture of softened kombu — remember, it is a seaweed! The "sliminess" disappears once cooked. Kombu will reduce the starchiness of beans, shorten their cooking time, and will also cut down on their lethal flatulence! Add kombu to leafy green vegetables such as turnip greens and kale, or add it to our recipes for Sherried Swiss Chard or Spinach with Roasted Garlic.

Nonfat Dry Milk

You can add the instant nonfat dry milk found in your local market to sauces, casseroles, and baked goods as well as to milk and yogurt to boost nutrient values substantially.   When reconstituted, nonfat dry milk is not a great substitute tastewise for skim milk, so we prefer to add it during cooking or prior to serving whenever possible. And here's why.

There are 100 calories in 1/4 cup of dry mix, 10 grams of protein and only 1 gram of fat. One-fourth cup of milk powder supplies, in addition, 40 percent of your RDAs for vitamin B12, 31 percent for calcium, and 29 percent for both potassium and riboflavin.

To modify your own baked recipes or casseroles to add nonfat dry milk, simply replace an equal portion of dry ingredients with milk. For baked goods, substitute one-eighth of a portion of dry milk for flour. For example, in 2 cups of flour, substitute 1/4 cup of dry milk for 1/4 cup of flour. For casseroles, add 1 tablespoon per serving. Fortify single servings of dairy products such as yogurt or skim milk with 1 tablespoon, and add 1/4 teaspoon per serving to yogurt-based sauces.

Nori

Also known as laver or sea lettuce, nori is the paper-thin dark green sheet of seaweed wrapped around your sushi roll. One sheet (a scant 2 grams) of nori provides 20 percent of your daily ration for B6, 27 percent for vitamin D, and 8 percent for iron.

Sold in 8" x 7" dry sheets in the Asian section of your supermarket, nori should be stored in an airtight container, where it will keep indefinitely. It has a nutlike flavor that, when lightly toasted, makes an excellent snack on its own. Crumbled and toasted, it blends invisibly into salads. Cut or torn, add it to stir-frys and casseroles; serve it crumbled over a baked potato, or as a garnish for rice and vegetable dishes. Nori is high in sodium, and thus should be avoided by those monitoring their diet for salt

Brewer's Yeast

Brewer's yeast is a nutritionally potent powder sold largely in health food stores. It is slightly more nutritious than the generic nutritional yeast you might find in the bulk bins in your health food store. One teaspoon (9 grams) supplies 100 percent RDA for thiamine, 88 percent for folacin, 24 percent for both copper and chromium, 21 percent for riboflavin, 13 percent for selenium and 11 percent for vitamin B6. For 25 calories, you can't beat that!

When sprinkled over salads or grains, it makes a great seasoning. Add it routinely to casseroles and stews. We even sprinkle it over popcorn with a little low-sodium soy sauce or vegetable broth to make it stick to the popcorn.

There are many brands of brewer's yeast with a wide range of flavors, so try several until you find the one you like best.

Shiitake Mushrooms

When added to any vegetable stir-fry, vegetarian pizza or stew, the meaty texture and wholesome flavor of shiitakes make for a hearty meal. In California and New York we can find fresh shiitakes in supermarkets. If you don't find them, ask your grocer to carry them. Look for dried shiitake mushrooms in the Asian section of your local market or order them from the company we recommend in Appendix A.

One large mushroom sports 70 calories and delivers 40 percent of your daily nutritional needs for potassium, 14 percent for niacin, and 6 percent for iron. In addition, this mushroom has 6 grams of fiber. Research in Japan indicates that shiitakes contain lentinan (a cancer-fighting substance), as well as a form of vitamin D (one of only a few vegetables that contain this nutrient).

They may be slightly more expensive than standard mushrooms, but a few go a long way. To soften the dried variety, soak them in hot water for 15 minutes. Squeeze dry, then trim off the stems and slice the caps evenly.

Soybeans

While you may not yet find the infamous soybean on your supermarket shelf, in the health food store countless soy products now replace traditional foods, including soy cheese, soy milk, ice cream, and soymeat hot dogs and bacon. Aside from tofu, the only soy product we use in this book is the bean itself. Nutritionally, soybeans are a good choles-terol-free replacement for meat, as they contain all essential amino acids. Thus, soy protein is high quality. Compare cooked soybeans to a cooked egg. The former is 11 percent protein while the egg is 13 percent. In addition, 14 grams, only 55 calories— only about10 beans — provides 20 percent of your daily needs for selenium and vitamin E, two very important antioxidants.

If you can't find soybeans in your health food store, order them by mail (see Appendix A). Again, a little goes a long way! While most cookbooks will tell you that soybeans take longer to cook than kidney, black, or lima beans, I haven't found that to be the case. So simply substitute a percentage of soybeans in any bean dish you are prepar-ing. Ten percent will fortify your meal substantially. Soybeans by them-selves have a fairly neutral flavor, and can thus invisibly be added to any recipe.

Tofu

Tofu is fresh soybean curd. It is made by coagulating, or curdling the white milk of soaked soybeans. Tofu is by far the most versatile of pro-tein foods in the world. It can be whipped as a sauce, stir-fried as a meat alternative, and even used for cheese in cheesecake or lasagne.

Nutritionally, compare the 80 calories and 10 grams of protein in a 3" x 2" piece of tofu (120 grams) with the 170 calories and 20 grams of protein in a similar serving of sirloin steak (120 grams or 4 oz.) For half the calories, you get 13 percent of your iron needs compared to 18 percent with steak, a close tie; and 13 percent of your requirements for calcium and phosphorus. Double the serving of tofu, by including it not only as an entree but in a tofu-based cream sauce and, for the same calories as in a single steak, but twice as much food, you will get as much protein as if you had eaten a steak plus the calcium and phos-phorus.

You will find tofu in both soft (for sauces) and firm (excellent grilled) varieties in the refrigerator section of most supermarkets. Check for the expiration date and buy the freshest tofu possible. If handled right, fresh tofu can be kept for up to a week in the refriger-ator. It should be kept submerged in cold water, and the water should be changed daily. Simply pour off the old and add fresh water. Nori is a brand name of tofu that is packaged airtight to keep without refrigeration. While the fresh is preferable, this is great to keep on hand for those unexpected guests and that impromptu serving of dip with raw vegetables!

Wheat Germ

Wheat germ is the nutrient-packed embryo of the wheat kernel. It is a super antioxidant, being rich in vitamin E; 1 tablespoon (23 calories), contains 36 percent of your daily requirements, and 13 percent of your daily recommendations for selenium. That same tablespoon also has 30 percent of your requirements for vitamin K and 23 percent for manganese. We sprinkle wheat germ over everything!

Raw wheat germ available in the refrigerator section in your health food store is the best. The commercial brand sold with cereals in supermarkets has been processed and has been sitting on that shelf for a very long time. The oil in wheat germ will go rancid. Once opened, store wheat germ in an airtight container in your refrigerator.

Add wheat germ to salads, soups, shakes, cereals, casseroles, sauces, just about everything!

GENERAL COOKING TIPS

Baking, Reducing Fat and Sugar

You may bake all kinds of foods, including desserts, on the Anti-Aging Plan, as long as you (1) start out with wholesome ingredients, meaning whole, unrefined, unprocessed grains, flours, etc.; and (2) apply what you have learned in this book about fats, oils, and sugars.

Most standard recipes for baking put great emphasis on observing exact measurements and proportions in order to obtain a successfully baked finished product. We disagree. We have experimented with reducing both the fat and the sugar content of any recipe, and have obtained delicious baked goods that taste at least as good as the sweeter, fattier original. Often modified recipes even taste superior, and they definitely digest better. So in addition to recommending baking recipes contained in this book, we recommend that you routinely reduce the fat/oil content and the sugar content of all of your baking recipes, to the degree that pleases your palate. You may find that you can go very far in reducing these. See, for example, our recipe for Chocolate Layer Cake(page 277).

Many commercially sold cake mixes, muffin mixes, even pancake mixes, now offer "Lite" and "No cholesterol" recipes (usually omitting the oil or eggs) as alternatives to the standard package directions. Always use these lighter recipes. Few brand-name baking mixes contain wholegrain flours, so we don't recommend using them often, but as occasional time-savers and cost-cutters, they are all right as long as you follow the "Lite" or "No Cholesterol" package directions.

Broccoli Stems; Preparing
In many of our recipes we use the thick, trunklike broccoli stems that many people are in the habit of discarding. They are luscious and nutritious, and here is a tip on preparing them for use: After removing and saving the broccoli flowerets, first slice the trunklike stem crosswise at its middle to check its interior. If the interior is totally dried-out woody fibers, then that stem is unusable — even cooking will not soften it — and should be discarded; the interior should look solid and still juicy and fresh. With a sharp knife, gently remove the tough outer skin from the broccoli stems. You may also pull any little tough leaves off the stem and cut off any discolorations or knobbly stubs.

Broths
Broths can be as instant as a bouillon cube, as recyclable as the cooking water from steamed greens or vegetables, or as nutritious as the water saved from soaking kombu seaweed or dried shiitake mushrooms (see references in this section). Instant broth cubes tend to be rather salty, although they are great in a pinch. The water you generally toss from steamed vegetables is both fragrant and flavorful. For a satisfying winter drink, add to this vegetable broth a little grated ginger, and a pinch of herbs. By far the most nutritious base for broth is the soak water left over from softening kombu or shiitake mushrooms. The Japanese use this regularly in their form of broth called dashi. Dashi will keep in the refrigerator for up to 5 days.

Here is a basic vegetable broth which, when prepared with half as much water, doubles as a low-fat between-meal soup.

For 1 gallon, or 16 cups of broth, fill a large kettle with 10 cups of water or dashi (see above). Bring to a boil. Add 4 large onions, quartered; 2 chunkily chopped green bell peppers, 2 large fresh tomatoes, quartered; 1 head cabbage, shredded; 1 bunch celery, chopped; and 2 carrots, sliced into bite-size pieces. Return to a gentle boil and simmer for 45 minutes.

As a soup, this pot makes 12 servings with 40 calories in each serving. To use as broth in the recipes for this book, simply remove the vegetables with a slotted spoon.

Chicken broth is as traditional as apple pie, only much simpler to make! For 1 gallon (freeze broth or use it as the cooking liquid to flavor grains): In a large kettle, heat 10 cups of water to a rolling boil. Add a skinned 4-to-5 pound chicken or a leftover turkey carcass and simmer, covered, for 2 hours. Add 8 celery ribs with leaves, 1/2 bay leaf, 1 small chopped onion, and 4 chopped carrots. Simmer another 30 minutes. Cool. As the stock cools, skim any remaining grease off the top with a heavy-weight paper towel fitted into a strainer.

Butter, Use of at the Table

You may notice that we do not use butter anywhere in this book. Margarine really does not fare much better in the fight against arteriosclerosis. But don't let that discourage you! There are many alternatives. Olive oil, while still 100 percent fat, is a healthier monounsaturated alternative. Use it — sparingly — over baked or mashed potatoes. Try apple butter on toast and bread. You will find apple butter — in fact many fruit butters, which are 100% pureed, unsweetened fruit — alongside peanut butters and jams. Pureed and seasoned soy or white bean pâté makes another creative and nutritious creamy butter to serve with rolls at the dinner table. Over vegetables, squeeze fresh lemon juice instead of the habitual butter. And finally, there is a synthetic alternative called Butterbuds available at most supermarkets.

Cauliflower Stems, Uses For

When using cauliflower, you may, after cutting off the flowerets for use in the recipe, save the stems and the heart of the cauliflower in the produce drawer of your refrigerator and then use them, thinly sliced or grated, in salads for a delicious and crunchy texture and taste.

Chicken and Turkey, Ground

In all recipes in which we suggest ground chicken, you can reduce the already low fat content of the ground chicken if you obtain it from a butcher and ask him to use only white meat with skin removed; and the same is true for ground turkey. Check the labels carefully for the fat content in commercially made ground poultry.

Cottage Cheese, Heating

See also "Cottage Cheese" in the Anti-Aging Glossary of Foods (page 286). Cottage cheese may be very slowly heated just before serving, but it must be closely watched. It should never be boiled, simmered, fried, or heated at a high temperature, or heated for a prolonged period of time because it will lump and separate into curds, watery liquids, and stringy filaments.

Deglazing

Deglazing of your cooking utensil is a particularly useful cooking technique in lowfat nutrient-rich cuisine. In our recipes, we often "dry-fry" (see the entry in this section for "Dry-Frying"). When you dry-fry, the foods will crisp and brown slightly and sometimes stick to the pan. The process of loosening them from the pan's cooking surface with all of their browned and crisped flavor is called deglazing. The best way to deglaze, and this is the method used by chefs of classic cuisines all over the world, is to pour in one or more jolts of any kind of beverage containing alcohol — wine, beer, sherry, marsala, etc. The alcohol-containing liquid instantly reacts with the glazed pan and the fried bits of food and they all unite into a flavorful beginning of a sauce. Remember that 85 percent of the calories and alcohol of the liquid that you add are burned off by the cooking process.

Dry Fry

To fry vegetables in their own juices, a good nonstick skillet is essential. Spray the skillet lightly with olive oil or add a teaspoon of broth, wine, or water before placing over the heat. Once the vegetables have been added, cover the skillet for a minute to discourage liquids from evaporating too quickly. Then, with a rubber spatula or wooden spoon, as the vegetables begin to stick to the pan, stir the brown bits from the bottom of the pan up into the stir (dry)-fry.

Add liquids sparingly as you cook the vegetables. To keep them from scorching, cover the skillet and stir frequently.

Egg Yolks, Leftover, Uses For

Many of our meganutrient recipes suggest the use of egg whites. Egg yolks are not recommended because 82 percent of the calories in yolks come from fat. However, one egg yolk supplies you with 18 percent of your daily requirements for vitamin B12. They do have some redeeming qualities, and are used as a meat alternative in many vegetarian recipes. The following dessert filling should be used sparingly.

Apple Custard Filling: 3 large apples, peeled and cored, juiced and grated rind of 1 lemon, 1/4 cup sugar, 1 tablespoon flour ,3 tablespoons water, 3 egg yolks, 1 teaspoon vanilla.

Grate the apples in a food processor. Combine the grated apple, lemon juice, lemon rind, and sugar in a saucepan. Heat over medium-high heat, uncovered, until almost boiling. Combine the flour with the water and add to the apples. Stir until the apples thicken. Lightly beat the egg yolks and whisk in a few tablespoons of the hot apple mixture. Pour the egg yolk mixture into the apples, stirring constantly. Return to low heat and heat 3 minutes longer, stirring constantly until the filling thickens. Remove from the heat and stir in the vanilla. Spoon 1/4 cup of this apple custard in between layers of Spiced Honey Cake (page 278) or serve one tablespoon per portion with Noodle Kugel (page 281). Calories per 1 tablespoon of Apple Custard Filling: 40.

Fish, Skinning

In recipes using fish, you can further reduce fat content by skinning the fish. It is difficult to skin raw fish, and also the skin does protect the delicate fish flesh during cooking, so we suggest that you remove fish skin after cooking, that is, just prior to eating. The skin will slip easily off still-warm cooked fish.

Ginger, Fresh, Preparing

In our recipes calling for fresh ginger, here is how we recommend preparing fresh ginger: Ginger is a root, with a thick outer skin. This should be peeled off with a small knife, removing any bulging knots. Holding a small grater over a plate, firmly press the ginger into the grater and brush up and down, grating as you would parmesan cheese.

Meats, Trimming
In recipes using any kind of meat, trim off all fat before cooking.

Nut Butters, Reducing the Oil In
The oil in the nut butter sesame tahini will usually separate from the nut paste and rise to the top of the container. If you want to reduce the fat content of a dish that uses tahini, you may pour off this separated oil from the tahini into a separate container (save it for other recipes that use sesame oil), and use just the dense nut paste in your recipe. You may need to soften up this dense paste in order to be able to mix it into a recipe. When you need to soften it up — in very small increments, while mashing constantly with a fork — add boiling water till the nut paste is moist enough so that you can mash it to a perfectly smooth consistency.

Note: This same principle applies to natural peanut butter— that is, the nonhydrogenated type — in which the peanut oil also separates from the peanut paste and rises to the top of the container.

Nuts, Toasting
For large amounts of nuts, spread in a shallow baking pan and bake in a preheated 350°F oven for about 10 minutes, stirring occasionally, until golden brown. Cool before chopping or processing.

For amounts of 1/2 cup or less, heat a medium-size dry skillet over medium heat. When hot, add the nuts and cook, shaking the pan frequently, until golden brown, about 6 minutes. Cool as above.

Oils, Refrigerating
We suggest that you refrigerate all liquid oils, which will otherwise become rancid rapidly. Since some oils become semisolid when refrigerated and will then not pour out of the usually long and narrow-necked containers that they are packaged in, you might want to keep a small amount of each of your oils in the refrigerator in a small, squat, wide-necked jar that you can fit a spoon or scoop into.

Cooking Oil Sprays, Safety Of
In most of our recipes, we recommend the use of the cooking oil sprays that are now commonly available in any supermarket. Please read carefully the warning on the spray container that tells you always to

spray the oil only onto a cold heating surface. Never spray it onto a heated pan, and never use it near a hot surface or a flame. This warning applies to any substance in a spray can.

Cooking Oil Sprays, Alternatives To
If you either cannot find cooking oil sprays, or do not want to spend the money on them, you may in some of our recipes use the following method, instead, to lubricate the cooking surface of a pan, or grease a baking pan, still using the absolute minimum of oil: Place 3 to 4 drops (more or less, depending on the size of the cooking utensil that needs to be lubricated) of oil onto the inner surface of the cooking utensil. Using your fingertips, rub the oil all over the cooking surface.

Peppers, Hot, Handling
A word of caution for whenever you handle any variety of hot peppers, such as jalapeño, habañero, serrano, and chile de arbol: The oils in these peppers are very powerful and lingering, and can irritate your skin. You should wear rubber gloves when you chop or seed or otherwise handle these peppers. Especially be careful not to touch or rub your eyes after handling hot peppers.

Peppers, Red, Roasting
Preheat the broiler. Cut the peppers in half, remove the seeds, and spread them out, cut side down, on a cookie sheet. Flatten them out by pressing them down with your hand. Put the peppers under the broiler for approximately 5 minutes, or until the skins blacken. Remove from the oven and place the peppers in a plastic bag. Twist shut and allow the peppers to "sweat" for 10 minutes. Remove from the bag and rub the blackened skins off, rinsing under cold running water if necessary to eliminate all the black bits.

Poultry, Skinning
In all of our recipes that use chicken, turkey, or any other poultry, we always mean skinned poultry. The skin is almost entirely fat, and it should be removed and discarded. As to whether to remove the skin of poultry before or after cooking, some recent research seems to indicate that leaving the skin on during cooking will not increase the fat content of the meat itself; however, for the purposes of the Anti-Aging

Plan, we suggest — to be on the safe side — that you remove all skin and pockets of fat from poultry before cooking. The added advantage of doing this is that whatever cooking liquids or broths are produced in the course of the recipe will not need to be defatted. Defatting stocks, broths, and pan drippings is a messy and time-consuming job (unless you are cooking a whole day in advance, which gives you time to refrigerate stock, broth, or drippings for 24 hours, then simply lift the cold, congealed fat off the top of the stock, broth, or pan drippings the following day).

Raisins, Plumping
There is a delicious way to plump up raisins for use in salads, or in desserts. These plumped up raisins are also excellent as a topping over ice cream, or in yogurt. Spread out 1/2 cup of raisins in a small, shallow bowl. Soak them in water-diluted vanilla extract till they absorb all of the extract. Any other extract, or another liquid such as a liqueur, may be substituted to plump the raisins.

Salt, Use of at the Table
We suggest freshly squeezed lemon juice over any of the foods that you would usually salt, from appetizers to main dishes to vegetables to almost anything. The potency of the lemon juice is similar to that of salt. Lemon juice will "marry" harmoniously with almost any food just as salt does.

Sauces, Reduction Method For
This is a low-fat way to obtain a thick sauce. "Reduction method" simply means that you simmer the sauce very slowly, for many hours, over the lowest possible heat, in an uncovered pan. In this way, you slowly boil away most of the water content of the sauce.

Seeds, Crushing, Cracking, or Grinding
In our recipes that use whole seeds which must be crushed or cracked, we suggest a mortar and pestle, but if you do not have one and are unable to find one locally, you may use a manual or small electric coffee grinder. Use it only for grinding or cracking herbs and spices, not coffee (because the powerful flavors will linger in the grinder).

Seeds, Dry Roasting

"Dry roasting," or toasting, brings out all the flavor of fennel seeds, sesame seeds, sunflower seeds, or any other seed you could mention. Place a small, heavy skillet over low heat until hot. Add your seeds and toast, shaking the pan occasionally, for several minutes until the seeds are fragrant and lightly colored. Cool, then use as is or grind to a coarse powder in a spice or coffee grinder. You can also crush the seeds in a mortar with a pestle or with the handle of a heavy knife.

Spinach, Washing

We use spinach in many of our recipes. Although frozen spinach is always substitutable and adequate, fresh spinach is the most delicious. The only thing that seems to make most people choose frozen spinach (besides unavailability of fresh) is that many people find spinach harder to wash than other green vegetables. It is very sandy, and how do you get out all that sand without bruising or disintegrating the tender, flavorful leaves? Here is our fast, effective, and yet gentle way of washing spinach:

Fill a large bowl or pot with cool water. Hold the bunch of spinach firmly by its roots and stems. Dunk the leaves into the water and swish gently a few times to dislodge the sand. Drain the water and repeat a second time with fresh water. Unless your spinach is extremely earthy, two dunks should suffice. Note: This washing method works for any delicate green that has tender leaves (such as basil).

Tomatoes, Peeling and Seeding

Easy! To peel fresh tomatoes, dip into boiling water for about 1 minute, or until the skins just begin to crack. Then, using a slotted spoon, plunge into cold water. The skin will now slip off easily. To seed, gently slice the tomato in half and, using a grapefruit spoon (a spoon with a serrated edge) or tomato knife, scrap out the seeds and membrane.

Vegetables, Roasting

Almost any vegetable can be roasted as an alternative to steaming, boiling, or baking. Roasting is definitely a desirable alternative to frying, and can produce a taste lusciously similar to frying if done properly (it is the slight blackening of the surface of the vegetable in roasting that approximates the fried flavor). We offer here the following general vegetable-roasting formula, which can be applied to a wide variety of vegetables such as zucchini and all kinds of other squashes, mushrooms, and so on.

Cut the vegetable into either strips or chunks or bite-sized pieces, depending on the vegetable and on what size piece you prefer. Spray a cookie sheet or baking pan with canola oil spray. Roast root vegetables separately from those grown above the ground; root vegetables have less water and will need longer to roast. Spread the vegetables on the sheet so that they do not overlap. Roast in a 375°F oven till the vegetables are cooked tender, approximately 5 minutes for above-ground vegetables and 30 minutes for root. Cherry tomatoes, mushrooms (stems removed), and eggplant blacken nicely.

For on the grill, place the vegetables about 3 inches above the hot coals.

Wheat Germ, Toasting
In recipes using wheat germ, we have not specified raw or toasted. This is a matter of taste. Raw wheat germ is a little more nutritious, but some people prefer the taste of toasted wheat germ. You may toast raw wheat germ in your toaster-oven or in a regular oven by spreading it out in a thin layer and baking at 325°F for approximately 5 minutes, watching over it carefully and stirring it once or twice, because wheat germ is very delicate, toasts quickly, and burns easily.

Yogurt, Heating
See also Yogurt in the Anti-Aging Glossary of Foods. Yogurt may be slowly heated just before serving, but it must be closely watched. It is delicate. It must never be boiled, simmered, fried, heated at a high temperature, or heated for a prolonged period of time because it will curdle. By "curdle" we mean that it will lose its smooth creaminess and will separate into solids and liquids. Even if it does curdle, however, its flavor will not be impaired.

TIPS FOR FREEZING

As an introduction to this section, we repeat what we have said elsewhere in the book about our Quantity-Cook-and-Freeze Option. Quantity-cooking a recipe so that it lasts for eight meals instead of one is not eight times as much work. On the contrary, it actually saves time, and money. It involves one shopping trip instead of seven, it uses the same number of pots and pans, and it is a savings on the use of the stove. Once you read the tips below, freezing will become easy for you. In addition, we have included freezing, thawing, and reheating instructions after each Megameal recipe. In today's world with microwave ovens and "freezer-to-oven-or-microwave" dishware, you can even freeze your portions in the same dishware on which you are going to serve them.

For average capacity freezers, we recommend that you maintain a stockpile of thirty-two carefully arranged frozen single-serving meals. If you are freezing for a family, see suggestions further in this chapter.

Your freezer temperature should be kept at 0° F.

Storing Your Frozen Meals

Plastic freezer-to-oven-or-microwave dishware is especially convenient in the oblong 1-pint size. These stack well and fit into a briefcase. We recommend that you wrap even these dishes in a baggie to insure against possible leakage.

Pyrex freezer-to-oven-or-microwave dishware is only appropriate if it features a sealable top.

Plastic freezer baggies. Especially sandwich sizes for single portions. Noodle dishes and quiches can easily be stored in larger freezer bags. These are an absolute must, as filled with Megameal dishes they will stack compactly into your freezer.

Freezer-safe plastic wrap. Waxed on one side, this works well to freeze burritos, bananas, and pizza. Foods should be well wrapped in several layers and sealed with electrical freezer, or surgical tape. Do not use regular waxed paper or plastic wrap.

Small plastic containers. Convenient for storing sauces such as pesto, tofu sesame sauce, or extra tomato paste.

Ice cube trays. Perfect for storing small amounts of pregrated fresh ginger, minced garlic, shredded cheese, or broths. Store the trays in large plastic freezer baggies.

Electrical, duct or surgical tape.   For labeling your meals by name and date of cooking. It adheres well in the freezer and washes clean. A ballpoint pen on a room-temperature surface is the best kind of marker. The most important part of the labeling is the date that the food was cooked.

It is most important that you list your freezer's contents. Attach a graph onto your freezer door. This is the easiest way to efficiently rotate your frozen meals and not lose the dishes in the rear.

Hygiene

It is good to wash your hands before handling and packaging foods for freezing. The harmful bacteria such as staphylococcus and salmonella can be transmitted from a raw food that you are about to cook to your hands, and then from your hands to a food that you are about to freeze.

The same is true of cutting boards and utensils; wash them after each usage, and before touching other foods to them.

Note that freezing does not kill bacteria. If microbial or enzymatic activities have begun on a food before you freeze it, the freezing will only temporarily arrest the process. Therefore, thaw your meals out in the refrigerator rather than overnight or all day long on the kitchen counter.

ABCs of Freezing

The four essential requirements for efficient and successful home freezing are:

A. *Initial quality.* Freeze only top-quality foods. Freezing retains quality and flavor; it cannot improve on them.

B. *Speed.* The quicker fruits and vegetables are frozen after picking, the better the frozen product will be. So do not let your produce sit in your refrigerator. It is preferable to shop fresh before cooking.

C. *Proper packaging.* Use food wraps designed especially for freezing; they're readily available at most food stores.

D. *Rapid cooling of foods before freezing.* In the anti-aging meal plan, you will most often be freezing cooked foods, so remember this tip: Set the cooking utensil (pot, loafpan), with the cooked food in it, in a pan of ice water. Place it in the refrigerator until cool. A general rule: food temperature must be lowered to below 40° F withhin 4 hours to reduce growth of bacteria.

After cooling, freeze your meal rapidly. You should place the food in the coldest part of the freezer. Space items out in your freezer to allow for some cold air circulation. The rear of the freezer compartment is slightly colder than the front (in a typical kitchen refrigerator). If time and space permit, do not stack foods to be frozen on top of foods that have already been frozen. Try instead to freeze packages in a single layer, leaving a 1" space between packages, just until they are solidly frozen — usually overnight — then you may stack them to save space. With a packed freezer, this might not be practical.

Most foods freeze well. Exceptions: Cooked egg whites and raw salad vegetables, such as lettuce and tomatoes, do not freeze well. There is a general concensus that potatoes do not freeze well. However, when they are part of a larger, moist dish, they tend to dry out less.

Depending on the method that you plan to use to reheat the frozen meals (oven, top of stove, or microwave), you may want to slightly undercook certain dishes, as they will undergo slight additional cooking when you reheat them. Reheating instructions follow each of our thirty Megameal recipes.

Freezing Meat, Fish, and Poultry

Wrap well in freezer-weight foil (or other heavy-duty wrapping material), forming it carefully to the shape of the contents. This expels air. Fold and crimp ends of the package to provide a good, lasting seal.

Limit freezing of fresh (unfrozen) meats or seafoods to 12 pounds at a time.

Always thaw meat in its freezer wrap. Don't refreeze meat that has completely thawed; meat, whether raw or cooked, can be frozen successfully only once.

Thawing

Frozen foods may be defrosted in the refrigerator, at room temperature, or by heating. Thawing at room temperature is the least recommended. Bacteria may grow as the outer layer of food defrosts.

Once thawed, frozen food spoils more rapidly than nonfrozen food, and must be refrigerated promptly and used soon after thawing.

Accidental Thawing

If a frozen portion of a One-A-Day Megameal should accidentally thaw before you want to use it, it may, under certain conditions, be safely refrozen. The process of thawing and refreezing doesn't make foods unsafe. As a general rule, food may be refrozen, if not completely thawed, or if thawed for only a very short time in the refrigerator. It should still feel cold to the touch and ice crystals should still be visible. It is generally less advisable to refreeze thawed fish, or other seafood, and casseroles.

Foods that have thawed slowly, over a period of several days, to a temperature above 40° F are not likely to be fit for refreezing. Meats, poultry, most vegetables, and some prepared foods may become unsafe to eat. Any unpleasant-looking or bad-smelling food should be discarded.

Freezing for a Family

Most of our One-A-Day Megameals are one-dish casserole type meals. When frozen in their entirety in one container these dishes benefit from special handling methods. If you are cooking for a family and maintaining a stockpile of meals, it will be easier for you to double the quantity of each recipe and freeze one whole recipe.

Generally, casserole-type dishes are best if they are frozen before baking. To bake frozen casseroles, place the casserole, unwrapped and uncovered, in a preheated oven while frozen or after partially thawing overnight in the refrigerator or after 3 hours at room temperature (casseroles should not be thawed entirely at room temperature due to the possibility of food poisoning).

Then bake your meal in the oven according to the recipe's instructions, or reheat in a covered sauce pan.

Freezer Burn

Freezer burn is defined as light-colored spots that appear on frozen foods, caused by loss of surface moisture due to faulty packaging or improper freezing methods. Foods with freezer burn can cause indigestion or even food poisoning and should be discarded.

Chapter 10
The Megameals

☀ *Classic Paella*

Serves 8

PAELLA IS ONE OF THOSE DISHES OFTEN ASSOCIATED WITH FANCY RESTAU-
RANTS, YET IT'S SIMPLE TO PREPARE. IN ADDITION TO THIS FIRST CLASSIC
PAELLA, WE WILL OFFER THREE VARIATIONS: A CLASSIC VEGETARIAN, A VEG-
ETABLE, AND A CHICKEN PILAF, WHICH IS THE PERSIAN OR TURKISH VERSION
OF PAELLA.

THE SECRET TO THIS CLASSIC IS THE TEXTURE OF THE RICE. UNDERCOOK
THE RICE THE FIRST TIME, AS IT WILL CONTINUE TO COOK WHEN YOU ADD THE
VEGETABLES, CHICKEN, AND FISH.

3 cups chicken broth (or use broth from the cooked chicken)
1 teaspoon cumin seeds
1 celery stalk with leaves, diced chunkily
2 1/2 cups brown rice
1/2 cup wild rice
1 3-pound skinned, boned, chicken,
     simmered for 1 hour and cut into bite-size pieces,
     or 2 1/2 cups cooked skinless chicken chunks
1 strip 3" x 1" kombu, soaked for 15 minutes and diced
1 medium-size red bell pepper, chopped fine
1 cup fresh or frozen peas
1/2 teaspoon dried oregano
1/3 cup white wine or additional broth (optional)
2 cloves garlic, pressed
1/2 teaspoon whole saffron
1/2 cup chopped fresh cilantro
Black pepper to taste
1 pound medium-size shrimp, shelled and deveined
16 mussels or clams, in shell, scrubbed

In a large heavy pot bring the broth to a gentle boil. Slowly add the
cumin seeds, celery, and rice. Cover and simmer over low heat for 25
to 30 minutes. The rice should be slightly undercooked.

Add the cooked chicken, kombu, red pepper, peas, and oregano.

Add a little white wine or broth if the rice is very dry. Cover and cook over low heat 5 minutes. Add the garlic, saffron, and cilantro. Stir, then add black pepper. Mix in the shellfish. Stir well, cover, and simmer for 5 minutes until the mussels or clams open.

To freeze: Line up your freezerware dishes and measure out your servings according to your needs, in single or family portions. Place immediately in your freezer. To thaw, leave your meal in the refrigerator overnight or when you leave for work in the morning. Reheat in the microwave or place in a double boiler over medium heat.

Calories per serving: 540. Percentage of calories from fat 10%, protein 44%, carbohydrates 45%, 215mg cholesterol.

Nutritional profile (% of RDA) per serving of Classic Paella: Vitamin A - 27, Vitamin C - 101, Vitamin D - 0, Vitamin E - 52, Vitamin K - 0, Thiamine - 50, Riboflavin - 17, Niacin - 30, Vitamin B6 - 29, Folacin - 24, Vitamin B12 - 0, Pantothenic Acid - 38, Biotin - 12, Calcium - 13, Phosphorus - 39, Magnesium - 48, Potassium - 33, Sodium - 2, Iron - 33, Copper - 44, Manganese - 51, Zinc - 27, Selenium - 53, Chromium- 62.

✳ *Classic Paella for Vegetarians*

Serves 8

IN THIS RECIPE, VEGETARIANS WILL HAVE TO JUGGLE A BIT TO MAKE UP FOR THE NUTRITIONAL VALUE FOUND IN THE SEAFOOD IN THE PRECEDING RECIPE FOR CLASSIC PAELLA, BUT IT CAN BE DONE IF THE SUGGESTIONS BELOW ARE FOLLOWED. NOTE THAT IT DIFFERS FROM THE FOLLOWING VEGETABLE PAELLA BOTH IN SEASONING AND IN THE PROTEIN SUBSTITUTIONS.

THIS RECIPE IS CONVENIENT FOR A FAMILY OR FOR COMPANY WITH MIXED MEAT AND VEGETARIAN PREFERENCES. SIMPLY, ONCE THE RICE IS PREPARED, SEPARATE THE RICE INTO TWO POTS AND PROCEED WITH MEAT IN ONE AND TOFU IN THE OTHER.

Prepare Classic Paella (as before), substituting 16 ounces firm tofu, cut into 1" cubes, for the chicken and seafood, adding it along with the kombu. At the same time add 3 tablespoons wheat germ, 4 teaspoons brewer's yeast, and a piece (5" x 2") of nori, torn into pieces.

Serve accompanied by broccoli and kale or turnip greens.
To freeze: Freeze as for Classic Paella.

Calories per serving: 375. Percentage of calories from fat 14%, protein 25%, carbohydrate 62%, 0 mg cholesterol.

❋ *Vegetable Paella*

Serves 8

ANY VEGETABLE COMBINATION COULD BE ADDED TO THIS PAELLA WHICH MAKES THIS A GREAT BASE-RECIPE WHEN YOU HAVE A REFRIGERATOR FULL OF VEGETABLES!

AN UNINFORMED VEGETARIAN DIET WILL DEFINITELY REDUCE CHOLESTEROL AND ANIMAL FAT INTAKE (NO BUTTER FAT), BUT IT CAN LEAD TO OTHER NUTRITIONAL DEFICIENCIES. YEAST AND SEAWEEDS CAN EASILY BE INCLUDED IN MOST RECIPES WITH VERY LITTLE ALTERATION TO FLAVOR IN ORDER TO BOOST THE B VITAMINS. TRY A NUMBER OF BRANDS OF BREWER'S YEAST. EACH ONE HAS A DISTINCTLY DIFFERENT FLAVOR. YOU MIGHT FIND ONE THAT WILL SATISFY ANY CRAVING YOU MAY HAVE FOR SALT!

TO SUPPLY ADEQUATE VITAMIN A, SERVE THIS PAELLA WITH STEAMED CARROTS, UNLESS CARROTS ARE USED AS A SUBSTITUTE FOR THE RED PEPPERS.

> 2/3 cup dried garbanzo beans (chickpeas),
>   soaked overnight and drained
> 1/2 cup dried soybeans, soaked with the garbanzos
> 1 teaspoon dried oregano
> 1/2 cup sunflower seeds
> 2 1/2 cups vegetable stock or water
> 4 teaspoons coriander seeds
> 2 cups brown rice
> 1 cup wild rice

2 strips (3" x 1") kombu,
    soaked for 15 minutes and chopped
6 cloves garlic, minced
1/4 cup low-sodium soy sauce
1/4 cup maple syrup
1/4 cup water
2 containers (16 ounces each) extra-firm tofu
2 cups frozen peas
Olive oil cooking spray
2 large red peppers, roasted (page 105)
    or 6 medium-size carrots, sliced into bite-size pieces
2 tablespoons brewer's yeast
1/2 cup fresh parsley, chopped
4 lemons, sliced

Preheat the oven to 350°F.

Cook the beans in a 2-quart saucepan for 10 minutes.

Drain the beans well. Sprinkle the oregano over the beans and stir. Spread the beans on an ungreased cookie sheet. Bake for 30 minutes, or until the beans crunch. When you hear them start to pop, like popcorn, it's time to take them out. At the same time that you are roasting the beans, roast the sunflower seeds on the rack above the garbanzo beans, or any way they will both fit your oven. Sunflower seeds only take 10 to 15 minutes — don't let them burn.

In a 3-quart saucepan, bring the vegetable stock or water to a boil. Add the coriander seeds and brown rice. Turn the heat down to low, and simmer, covered, for 15 minutes. Add the wild rice and kombu.

Stir 2 cloves of the garlic, the soy sauce, maple syrup, and 1/4 cup water together in a medium bowl. Slice the tofu into 1-inch squares and toss gently in the marinade. For a stronger flavor, leave the tofu in the marinade for 20 minutes or longer.

Cook the peas according to package directions.

Meanwhile, spray a small nonstick skillet with olive oil. Lightly stir-fry the remaining garlic cloves, and, if you are using carrots instead of red peppers, add the carrots with a little bit of water or broth. Cook briefly, 5 minutes.

When the rice has cooked a total of 30 minutes and is still a little crunchy, stir all the ingredients (including the brewer's yeast) together. The key to good paella is in the texture of the rice. If it's mushy, your flavors will all run together. Reheat over a low flame, or bake in a 350°F oven for 20 minutes.

Before serving, top with fresh parsley. Serve with sliced lemons.

To freeze: Follow freezing instructions for Classic Paella.

Calories per serving: 496. Percentage of calories from fat 25%, protein 33%, carbohydrates 24%, 0 mg cholesterol.

Nutritional profile (% of RDA) per serving of Vegetable Paella:
Vitamin A - 31, Vitamin C - 102, Vitamin D - 40, Vitamin E - 67, Vitamin K - 27, Thiamine - 113, Riboflavin - 32, Niacin - 41, Vitamin B6 - 141, Folacin - 72, Vitamin B12 - 80, Panthothenic Acid - 55, Biotin - 22, Calcium - 16, Phosphorus - 49, Magnesium - 69, Potassium - 48, Sodium - 6, Iron - 51, Copper - 54, Manganese - 63, Zinc - 31, Selenium - 72, Chromium - 36.

✳ *Chickpea or Chicken Pilaf*

Serves 8

PERSIANS AND TURKS CALL THEIR VERSION OF PAELLA "PILAF." IN THIS PILAF, MILLET IS THE HIDDEN TREASURE. IN THE REALM OF GRAINS, MILLET RANKS HIGH. ITS LIGHT, NUTTY FLAVOR AND SMOOTH TEXTURE MAKE IT A GREAT ALTERNATIVE TO RICE. MILLET HAS TWICE AS MUCH FIBER AS BROWN RICE, AND 25 PERCENT MORE PROTEIN. THIRTY PERCENT OF ITS CALORIES DO COME FROM FAT. HOWEVER, IF USED AS A BASE IN A CASSEROLE SUCH AS THIS, THE BALANCE OF LEAN VEGETABLES AND MEATS WILL MAKE UP FOR ITS ADDED RICHNESS.

THIS DISH CAN BE ADAPTED FOR A VEGETARIAN DIET BY SIMPLY SUBSTITUTING FIRM TOFU OR GARBANZO BEANS (CHICKPEAS) FOR THE CHICKEN.

Pilaf
Olive oil cooking spray
4 cloves garlic, minced
2 jalapeño chilies, seeded and minced
1 3/4 pounds skinless, boneless chicken breast,
    cut into bite-size pieces
    or 1 3/4 pounds firm tofu
    or 2 cups cooked garbanzo beans
1/2 pounds fresh shiitake mushrooms, chopped
31/2 cups broth or water, plus additional as needed
2 cups millet
1/4 cup wheat germ
2 red bell peppers, seeded and chopped
2 pounds mung bean sprouts
2 medium-size sweet potatoes, peeled and cut into 1/4" slices
3 sheets (each 4" x 2") nori, torn into pieces
Soy sauce or Tabasco sauce, to taste
1/2 cup fresh parsley, chopped
10 scallions, whites only, chopped

Spray a large non-stick skillet with olive oil and place over medium heat. Add the garlic and jalapeño peppers. Stir for 2 minutes. Add the chicken and quickly sear to seal in the flavor. Remove the chicken and set aside. Add the shiitake mushrooms. Add a little water or broth as needed to lightly stir-fry the mushrooms.

In a 3-quart saucepan, bring 3 1/2 cups of broth or water to a boil. Add the millet, wheat germ, red peppers, and chicken-shiitake-jalapeño-garlic mixture. Return to a gentle boil. Lower the heat, cover, and simmer for 20 minutes.

During the last 5 minutes of cooking, return the skillet to the stove. Add the bean sprouts, sweet potatoes, and nori. A touch of water will prevent the skillet from drying out; the moisture from the bean sprouts will then cook the vegetables. Stir-fry for 6 to 7 minutes. Drizzle in a little soy sauce or Tabasco to taste.

Add the bean sprout mixture to the millet mixture, along with the parsley and scallions.

Heat the cream sauce (below) in a saucepan until warm, then pour equally over each serving and offer extra hot sauce and additional chopped scallions if desired at the table.

Cream Sauce
3 cups packed fresh spinach with stems, washed
1 1/2 cups nonfat yogurt
1/4 cup nonfat dry milk
3 tablespoons dijon mustard
2 tablespoons grated onion
1 teaspoon dried thyme or tarragon
1/2 teaspoon white pepper
Buttermilk or nonfat (skim) milk

Steam the spinach for 4 minutes. Place the spinach in a food processor or blender with all of the remaining ingredients and puree until very creamy. For a thinner sauce, add buttermilk or nonfat milk. Set aside, covered.

For Vegetarians: Marinate 1 3/4 pounds cubed tofu in the marinade for Vegetable Paella. Stir the marinaded tofu in with the bean sprouts. Or add 2 cups cooked garbanzo beans along with the bean sprouts instead of the chicken.

To freeze: Simply portion out your servings into freezerware or freezer baggies. Place into the freezer as soon after cooking as possible. To thaw, place in the refrigerator overnight and reheat in the microwave or in a double boiler.

Calories per Serving: 584, Percentage of calories from fat 9%, protein 30%, carbohydrates 60%, 72 mg cholesterol.

Nutritional profile (% of RDA) per serving: Vitamin A - 229, Vitamin C - 215, Vitamin D - 54, Vitamin E - 71, Vitamin K - 100, Thiamine - 68, Riboflavin - 68, Niacin - 86, Vitamin B6 - 215, Folacin - 52, Vitamin B12 - 145, Pantothenic Acid - 57, Biotin - 20, Calcium - 32, Phosphorus - 63, Magnesium - 76, Potassium - 117, Sodium - 29, Iron - 69, Copper - 34, Manganese - 95, Zinc - 31, Selenium - 59, Chromium - 74.

✳ Super Burrito

Serves 8

Much like the tostada but more portable, the burrito is the ideal alternative to a classic sandwich. These are very easy to freeze. I prefer to use whole-wheat chapatis, because they are big and easy to roll. But if these are unavailable, or if you prefer corn tortillas, use them, by all means. The corn tortillas will dry out a little in the freezer. If possible, steam them to reheat, or they may crack. Pita pockets freeze well also.

When you make these burritos, double the recipe for the beans and freeze for later use.

Another time saver is to use cooked canned black beans. Cooked canned soybeans are available in some health food stores. Because soybeans boost the nutritional value of the meal by almost 25 percent, they must be included in order for this recipe to qualify as a One-A-Day Megameal. The kombu can be added, once soaked, to pre-cooked beans. When boiling the beans, the fragrance of the kombu may dominate your kitchen. The taste, however, once the beans are cooked and pureed, is invisible.

Filling

2 1/2 cups dried black beans, soaked overnight and drained
1 1/2 cups dried soybeans, soaked with the black beans
12 cloves garlic, peeled
6 jalapeño chiles, seeded and chopped
    or 1 dried Santa Fe chile, soaked, seeded, and chopped
    1/2 ounce (2 pieces 4" x 2") kombu, soaked for
    15 minutes and chopped
2 pounds skinless, boneless chicken breast,
    or 2 pounds swordfish, halibut, or other fish steak
Olive oil cooking spray
5 teaspoons ground cumin
1 tablespoon coriander seed
1 cup prune juice or broth
Dried hot pepper flakes (optional)
3 cups chopped cucumber
2 cups chopped fresh cilantro

Marinade for Fish
1/2 cup lemon juice
1/4 cup rice vinegar
2 tablespoons capers
Pinch of tarragon

Salsa
1 1/2 cups fresh or frozen corn
2 red bell peppers, chopped fine
1 green bell pepper, chopped fine
10 large scallions, whites only, chopped
1 teaspoon ground chili powder (optional)
1/2 red onion, minced

8 whole-wheat chapatis or corn tortillas

Place both beans, the garlic, chilies, and kombu in a 3-quart saucepan with enough water to cover. Bring to a boil, reduce the heat, and simmer for 45 minutes, or until the beans are tender. Puree the beans with their liquid in a food processor or mash with a fork or potato masher.

Meanwhile, marinate the fish, if using, in mixture of lemon juice, vinegar, capers, and tarragon for 30 minutes.

To make the refried beans: Generously spray a nonstick skillet with olive oil. Add the pureed beans and place over medium heat. Mix in the cumin and coriander seed. If you like spicy beans, you might want to add some dried hot pepper flakes (we do). Stir the beans frequently, turning the batter from the bottom to the top. In a good nonstick skillet it will turn crusty without sticking. As the liquid in the beans begins to dry up, slowly add the prune juice, 1/4 cup at a time. Slowly "refry" the beans for 15 minutes.

Place the chicken on a rack in a broiler pan. Broil 3 to 4 inches from the heat, turning to brown both sides, about 10 minutes total cooking time. Or, if you are making fish burritos, broil the marinated fish approximately 6 minutes for a 1" steak. Cool the cooked chicken or fish, then shred. Mix with the cucumber and cilantro and set aside.

To make the salsa: Spray a nonstick skillet with olive oil. Add the corn, red and green peppers, scallions and chili powder. Cover and cook over low heat for 5 minutes, or until the peppers are cooked crisp, not soft. Stir often. Remove from heat and stir in the red onion.

Spoon a rounded 1/3 cup of beans into each chapati. Follow with the meat, and a generous serving of salsa. Carefully roll the burrito up as tightly as possible. If any filling falls out during the rolling, stuff it back in.

Serve with extra salsa.

To freeze: These burritos can be prepared in their tortillas and wrapped tightly in freezer wax paper and stored in individual baggies. Or you can freeze filling in freezerware and prepare the burritos with fresh tortillas or chapatis. To do this, soften the tortillas by sprinkling them with a little water and steaming them in the microwave for a few seconds.

The salsa should be prepared fresh for each meal.

Calories per serving: 517. Percentage of calories from fat 15%, protein 32%, carbohydrates 53%, 55 mg cholesterol.

Nutritional profile (% of RDA) for 1 serving with chicken, with 1/2 cup of salsa: Vitamin A - 48, Vitamin C - 157, Vitamin D - 40, Vitamin E - 43, Vitamin K - 72, Thiamine - 91, Riboflavin - 32, Niacin - 56, Vitamin B6 - 86, Folacin - 84, Vitamin B12 - 62, Pantothenic Acid - 57, Biotin - 24, Calcium - 14, Phosphorus - 52, Magnesium - 68, Potassium - 87, Sodium - 32, Iron - 45, Copper - 26, Manganese - 66, Zinc - 26, Selenium - 88, Chromium - 45.

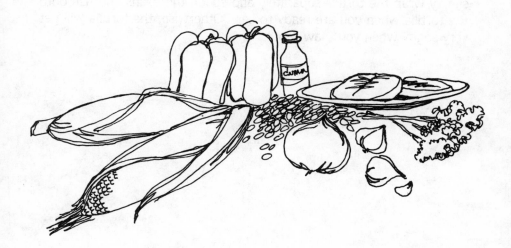

✳ *Tostada*

Serves 4

WHILE THE BASICS FOR THIS DELECTABLE DISH CAN BE FROZEN, WITH THE FRESH SALSA, ORANGES, CUCUMBER, AND TORTILLA ADDED AT THE TABLE, I RECOMMEND THAT THE SEAFOOD BE PREPARED FRESH FOR EACH SERVING. THE TENDERNESS OF FRESH FISH MATCHES THE HEARTINESS OF THE BEANS. THEY ARE CALORICALLY LOW, SO ENJOY THEM BOTH.

FRESH SALSA ALWAYS ADDS LIFE TO A TOSTADA, BUT A GOOD, OIL-FREE COMMERCIAL SALSA WILL DO JUST AS WELL. COMMERCIAL CANNED SOY AND BLACK BEANS ARE ALSO AVAILABLE.

Prepare the recipe for Super Burritos, but assemble as follows:

Layer each warm tortilla with 1/3 cup refried beans, spread into a smooth base. Circle the perimeter with peeled, thinly sliced cucumber and fresh orange sections. Cover the center with shredded iceberg lettuce and spoon on some Fresh Salsa (recipe below). Top the masterpiece with the hot swordfish, and garnish with a few extra orange sections.

To freeze: If you choose to freeze both the beans and the fish, then layer each freezerware dish with a serving of beans, then a strip of freezer plastic, followed by the serving of fish. This way, the fish can easily be separated from the beans after you defrost both. The layering of tortilla, beans and fish is important, so that flavors do not merge together.

Use fresh chapatis or tortillas. If you are taking this dish to work, simply wrap the tortilla separately and spoon the beans and fish onto the tortilla when you are ready to eat. Otherwise, the tortilla will get very soggy when you thaw it out.

❋ *Fresh Salsa* ❋

Makes about 2 cups

1 bunch fresh cilantro
3 red bell peppers, roasted (page 105) and chopped
3 fresh tomatoes, chopped and drained
1 1/2 cups chopped onions

Tear off (or snip off with scissors) all the cilantro leaves. Wash gently but thoroughly and chop coarsely. Mix with the roasted peppers, tomatoes, and onions in a bowl and store in the refrigerator until serving time. The salsa can be prepared several hours earlier.

Calories per 1/2 cup serving of salsa: 31. Percentage of calories from fat 5%, protein 15%, carbohydrate 79%, 0 mg cholesterol.

Calories per serving (1 tostada): 500, Percentage of calories from fat 21%, protein 31%, carbohydrates 47%, 31mg cholesterol.

Nutritional profile (% of RDA) for One Tostada with 1/2 cup salsa:
Vitamin A - 56, Vitamin C - 120, Vitamin D - 40, Vitamin E - 41, Vitamin K - 112, Thiamine - 80, Riboflavin - 25, Niacin - 28, Vitamin B6 - 54, Folacin - 80, Vitamin B12 - 55, Pantothenic Acid - 35, Biotin - 19, Calcium - 12, Phosphorus - 50, Magnesium - 50, Potassium - 87, Sodium -30, Iron - 40, Copper - 26, Manganese - 66, Zinc - 27, Selenium - 66, Chromium - 27.

❋ *Vegetarian Burritos*

Serves 8

VEGETARIANS WHO WANT TO ENJOY THE SUPER BURRITOS SHOULD PRE-PARE SUPER BURRITOS (ABOVE), BUT OMIT THE CHICKEN AND STIR INTO THE BEANS PRIOR TO PUREEING 1 CUP COOKED SOYBEANS, 4 TEASPOONS BREWER'S YEAST, 4 PIECES (4" X 2")EACH KOMBU AND NORI, 3 TABLESPOONS WHEAT GERM, AND 1/2 CUP NONFAT DRY MILK.

THE KOMBU AND NORI FEED YOU WITH VITAMIN B-6, THE WHEAT GERM INCREASES BOTH ANTIOXIDANTS SELENIUM AND VITAMIN E BY 55 PERCENT. WITHOUT THE YEAST, THE B VITAMINS THIAMINE AND RIBOFLAVIN ARE WELL BELOW 50 PERCENT. THE NONFAT DRY MILK PROVIDES THE ONLY ACCESS TO THE ALL-IMPORTANT VITAMIN B-12 AND BOOSTS CALCIUM LEVELS.

IN PLACE OF THE CHICKEN DRY-FRY 1 LARGE "MEATY" SHIITAKE MUSH-ROOM PER PERSON.

To freeze: Follow the freezing instructions for Super Burritos.

Calories per serving: 564. Percentage of calories from fat 27%, protein 40, carbohydrate 28%, 1 mg cholesterol.

✳ *Mu Shu Chicken Or Tofu*

Serves 8

MU SHU, A CHINESE STUFFED PANCAKE, IS VERY SIMILAR IN CONCEPT TO THE MEXICAN BURRITO.

IF YOU LOVE CHINESE FOOD BUT FIND THAT IT IS USUALLY TOO SALTY OR TOO OILY, HERE IS A LIGHTENED YET JUST AS FLAVORFUL VERSION OF THE STANDARD MU SHU DISH. THESE ARE WONDERFUL, LIGHT, CHICKEN OR TOFU AND VEGETABLE-FILLED PANCAKES THAT ARE FUN TO EAT. BECAUSE CLASSIC, PAPER THIN MANDARIN PANCAKES ARE DIFFICULT TO MAKE (THEY ARE AVAILABLE IN THE FREEZER SECTION OF ORIENTAL MARKETS), WE RECOMMEND THAT YOU SUBSTITUTE WHOLE WHEAT CHAPATIS OR WHEAT TORTILLAS. THEY ARE A LITTLE HEAVIER, BUT THEY FREEZE MORE EASILY, AND ARE AVAILABLE WITH NO OIL.

ONCE THE VEGETABLES ARE CHOPPED, THIS MEAL COOKS UP IN 20 MINUTES.

THERE ARE A FEW TRADITIONAL CHINESE SPECIALTY INGREDIENTS I'VE INCLUDED IN THIS RECIPE; THEY ARE ALL OPTIONAL. WOOD EARS, FOR EXAMPLE, OR TREE EARS, OR MOOK YEE, AS THEY ARE TRADITIONALLY CALLED, ARE A MEMBER OF THE MUSHROOM FAMILY: WRINKLED AND DARK, THEY ARE NEUTRAL IN TASTE BUT ADD A CRISP AND EXOTIC TEXTURE TO THE DISH. IF YOU OMIT THESE INGREDIENTS AND MAKE THE RECIPE SIMPLY WITH THE FRESH VEGETABLES, YOU HAVE A MU SHU DISH THAT IS CRUNCHY, LIGHT, AND ESPECIALLY GOOD IN THE SPRING OR SUMMER. IF YOU WANT TO FOLLOW THE RECIPE TO THE LETTER TO BE MORE TRADITIONAL, YOU WILL BE ABLE TO FIND THESE INGREDIENTS IN ORIENTAL MARKETS OR IN THE ASIAN SECTION OF YOUR SUPERMARKET.

HOISIN SAUCE, A SPICY, SWEET, KETCHUP-LIKE CONDIMENT MADE FROM SOYBEANS, VINEGAR, SUGAR, WHEAT FLOUR, WATER, GARLIC, SESAME SEEDS, CHILI AND SPICES, IS ALSO READILY AVAILABLE IN MARKETS. BUT SINCE OUR RECIPE IS A CREATIVE AND HIGHLY NUTRITIOUS VERSION MADE WITH BLACK BEANS, WE STRONGLY SUGGEST THAT YOU MAKE IT AND, IN FACT, MAKE A DOUBLE OR TRIPLE RECIPE BECAUSE, ONCE IT IS IN YOUR REFRIGERATOR, YOU WILL FIND A THOUSAND OTHER USES FOR IT. HOISIN SAUCE SHOULD BE STORED IN A GLASS JAR.

YOU MAY PREFER TO FREEZE ONLY HALF THE RECIPE AND FREEZE THE OTHER HALF TO SERVE LATER OVER RICE. BUT THIS DISH IS SO GOOD FRESH THAT YOU'LL WANT TO HAVE A PARTY AND SERVE THE WHOLE THING!

8 whole-wheat chapatis or
   wheat tortillas or 16 mu shu pancakes

<u>Chicken and/or Tofu Marinade</u>
1/2 cup mirin (Japanese rice wine)
1/2 cup low-sodium soy sauce
1/2 cup chicken or vegetable broth
3 tablespoons peeled and grated fresh ginger
4 cloves garlic, minced
1 tablespoon honey
1/2 teaspoon sesame oil
1 pound skinless, boneless chicken breast,
   cut into bite-size pieces or 1 pound firm tofu, cubed

<u>Filling</u>
Olive oil cooking spray
3 tablespoon fresh ginger, minced
6 cloves garlic, minced
2 cups thin diagonal slices bok choy,
   leaves separated from stalks
2 cups thin diagonal slices kale
1 red bell pepper, seeded and thinly sliced
1 green bell pepper, seeded and thinly sliced
8 dried shiitake mushrooms, soaked for 15 minutes,
   then drained (saving broth) and chopped
2 cups mung bean sprouts
5 carrots, grated
1/4 cup dried wood ears, soaked 15 minutes
   with mushrooms and chopped (optional)
16 scallions, trimmed of green

<u>Hoisin Sauce</u>
1 cup cooked black beans (canned or freshly cooked)
1/4 cup wheat germ
1/3 cup brown rice vinegar or regular rice vinegar
1/4 to 1/3 cup honey
3 cloves garlic, quartered
2 tablespoon mirin (Japanese rice wine) or sweet sherry

2 tablespoon grated orange peel
1 tablespoon low-sodium soy sauce
1 teaspoon chili paste or 1/2 teaspoon Tabasco, or to taste
1/2 teaspoon ground star anise
1/2 teaspoon ground cloves
1/2 teaspoon ground cinnamon

Make a marinade by stirring the mirin, soy sauce, broth, ginger, garlic, honey and sesame oil in a flat baking dish. Add the chicken or tofu and marinate for 30 minutes.

Spray a large wok or skillet with olive oil. Place over a medium heat and, when hot, add the ginger and garlic and stir-fry for 1 minute. Add the bok choy stems and kale, cover, and cook over a medium flame for several minutes, stir, then cook for 1 more minute. Add a little mushroom broth if the bok choy sticks. Remove the chicken (or tofu) pieces from the marinade with a slotted spoon and add, along with the bell peppers, shiitake mushrooms, bok choy leaves and bean sprouts. Stir-fry for 3 minutes. Add the chicken marinade with the carrots and wood ears. Simmer for another 3 minutes, stirring often. The vegetables should be crisp, not soggy, especially if you plan to freeze and reheat later.

Place the chapatis or tortillas, wrapped in foil, in a warm oven (150°) or in your toaster oven at the lowest setting, just to warm them till serving time.

Broil the scallions in a broiler pan for 1 minute.

Puree all the ingredients for the hoisin sauce together in a food processor until creamy. Adjust spiciness to taste.

With a slotted spoon, transfer the chicken (or tofu) and vegetable mixture to a serving platter. Spread hoisin sauce over each warmed chapati or tortilla, add 1/3 cup or so of filling, top with broiled scallions, and roll up into a tight "burrito." If you are using the traditional delicately thin Chinese mu shu pancake, divide your 1/3 cup of filling in half to fill two thin pancakes and call that your individual serving. These can be a little messy, so have plenty of napkins.

To freeze: Mu shus are a little messy, so prepare for freezing over a sink! You may either prepare each pancake individually, wrap it tightly in freezer wax paper and store in freezer baggies, or store the filling in freezerware dishes and prepare the pancakes fresh for each serving.

The chapatis will be soggy if you prepare the mu shu individually. However, this may be more convenient for you. To thaw, place the mu shu in the refrigerator overnight. Reheat in the microwave or remove the wax paper and place them in a baking dish. Place in an oven pre-heated to 350° F and bake for 15 minutes.

Calories per serving (with chicken): 303, percentage of calories from fat 8%, protein 30%, carbohydrates 61%, 33 mg cholesterol.

Nutritional profile (% of RDA) per serving: Vitamin A - 177, Vitamin C - 165, Vitamin D - 13, Vitamin E- 39, Vitamin K - 58, Thiamine - 38, Riboflavin - 25, Niacin - 48, Vitamin B6 - 65, Folacin - 33, Vitamin B12 - 33, Pantothenic Acid - 28, Biotin - 8, Calcium - 17, Phosphorus - 43, Magnesium - 24, Potassium - 67, Sodium - 25, Iron - 31, Copper - 9, Manganese - 36, Zinc - 17, Selenium - 57, Chromium - 40.

✳ Chile Rellenos with Refried Beans

Serves 4

Yes, you can have all the exotic, cheese-stuffed Mexican foods, only now we have streamlined them so you can enjoy their rich taste without overdoing it calorically. This unusual creation was a duet with our computer. To maximize the nutritional value of chiles rellenos, we came up with this novel asparagus sauce. The Anaheim or Santa Fe chiles we use here are approximately 5 inches long. While they are milder than jalapeño chiles, their seeds should be removed before roasting. Don't use dried peppers, they will not stay firm enough to stuff. They take a little time to roast, but they are well worth it. Our recommended normal portion is 2 stuffed chiles per person with the accompanying refried beans, salsa, and asparagus sauce.

Stuffed Chiles
8 Anaheim chiles, seeded and roasted
1/2 cup low-fat or nonfat ricotta cheese
1/2 cup grated low-fat or nonfat Monterey jack
1/2 red bell pepper, roasted
   with the chiles (see above), then chopped
1/2 cup fresh or frozen corn kernels, thawed if frozen
2 tablespoons chopped fresh cilantro leaves
4 egg whites
1 tablespoon whole wheat flour

Refried Beans
1 1/2 cups dried pinto beans, soaked overnight and drained
1/2 cup dried soybeans, soaked with the pinto beans
1 large onion, chopped
2 teaspoons dried hot pepper flakes
8 cloves garlic, coarsely chopped
2 strips (3" x 1") kombu, soaked and chopped
2 sheets (4" x 2") nori
1 sweet potato, scrubbed and finely diced
2 teaspoons ground cumin

1 tablespoon brewer's yeast
Asparagus Sauce (page 247)
Salsa (optional)

Preheat the oven to 350°F.

Prepare the beans: In a 3-quart saucepan cover the presoaked and drained beans with fresh water. Add the onion, pepper flakes, and garlic. Bring to a boil, reduce the heat, and simmer until beans are tender, approximately 1 hour. Add the kombu while the beans are cooking. Puree the beans with their liquids in a food processor or mash with a fork or potato masher.

Spray a large nonstick skillet with olive oil. Add the beans, nori, sweet potato, cumin, and brewer's yeast. Heat slowly, stirring with a rubber spatula. The mixture will dry out, and a rich crust will form in the pan. Keep turning this crust over, mixing it into the beans. This is the "refry" part. The sweet potatoes remain slightly crunchy, adding texture.

For the stuffing, mix the cheeses, bell pepper, corn, and cilantro together in a medium-size bowl. Gently slice one end of each roasted chile from top to bottom. Spoon into each chili 1 heaping tablespoon of cheese stuffing. Press each chili closed and into its original long, thin shape.

Whip the egg whites until soft peaks form. While beating, slowly add the flour until stiff peaks form. Gently dip each stuffed chili into egg whites, covering from top to bottom. Lay side by side in an oiled baking pan. Bake for 30 minutes, or until golden brown.

n a small, heavy saucepan gently heat the asparagus sauce, stirring frequently. Adjust the seasonings.

Serve with the refried beans, and salsa if desired. Generously ladle asparagus sauce over the chili rellenos.

To freeze: Carefully place 2 chiles per serving into freezerware dishes. Ladle asparagus sauce over each. The egg white will lose its light appearance once frozen, so we suggest that each chile be completely covered with sauce. To thaw, place the dish in the refrigerator overnight and reheat in the microwave or in the oven preheated to 350°F for 15 minutes.

Calories in 2 stuffed rellenos: 531. Percentage of calories from fat 19%, protein 29%, carbohydrates 52%, 22 mg cholesterol.

Nutritional profile (% of RDA) per serving: Vitamin A - 133, Vitamin C - 160, Vitamin D - 74, Vitamin E - 83, Vitamin K -174, Thiamine - 239, Riboflavin - 80, Niacin - 48, Vitamin B6 - 200, Folacin - 195, Vitamin B12 - 140, Pantothenic Acid - 93, Biotin - 37, Calcium - 42, Phosphorus - 77, Magnesium - 66, Potassium - 112, Sodium - 28, Iron - 66, Copper - 51, Manganese - 57, Zinc - 43, Selenium - 61, Chromium - 103.

✳ *Stuffed Peppers*

Serves 8

MANY VEGETABLES CAN EASILY BE STUFFED. TRY TOMATOES, ZUCCHINI, POTATOES, AND EGGPLANT; AND THEY ALSO MAKE AN ELEGANT PRESENTATION AT THE DINNER TABLE. BELL PEPPERS ARE AN EASY WAY TO START, AS THEY HOLD TOGETHER WELL.

8 large green or red bell peppers

Rice
2 cups chicken or vegetable broth
1 cup brown rice
3 cloves garlic, minced
1 teaspoon dried oregano
1/2 teaspoon black pepper

Stuffing
1/2 teaspoon olive oil
3 cloves garlic, minced
1 pound ground turkey or 10 ounces firm tofu, cubed
4 medium-size fresh tomatoes, chopped
2 cups frozen corn kernels, thawed
1 can (8 ounces) kidney beans,

or 1/2 cup dried, soaked overnight and cooked till tender
4 sheets (4" x 2") nori, cut fine
2 teaspoons dried oregano
2 teaspoons dried tarragon
1 teaspoon black pepper or 1/2 teaspoon red pepper
1 cup low-fat or nonfat cottage cheese
Canola oil cooking spray

Preheat the oven to 350°F.

In a 2-quart saucepan, bring the chicken broth to a boil. Add the rice, garlic, oregano, and black pepper. Reduce heat to a simmer and cover. Simmer for 40 minutes.

Meanwhile, carefully cut out the stems and the surrounding 1/2" or so of the pepper so that you have a "lid" to put back on the pepper. The opening in the top should be big enough to clean and stuff the pepper. Carefully remove inner whitish membranes and the seeds without damaging the shell. Save the pepper lids. Rinse out the peppers with cold water to remove any remaining seeds.

To make the stuffing, heat the olive oil in a medium-size skillet over a low flame. Add the garlic and ground turkey (or cubed tofu), stirring lightly to cook evenly. While the turkey is still barely pink and tender, add the tomatoes. Cook over low heat for 5 minutes. Add the corn, kidney beans, nori, herbs, and pepper. Simmer for 3 minutes. Add the cooked rice and remove from the heat. Gently mix the cottage cheese into the stuffing.

Fill each pepper right up to the top, and replace the lid. Lightly spray an 8" x 8" baking dish with canola oil. Carefully stand peppers up, side by side in the dish. Bake for 30 minutes.

To freeze: This dish is one of the easiest to freeze. Simply place each pepper in either a freezerware dish or a freezer baggie. To thaw, place it in the refrigerator overnight and reheat in the microwave or in a covered baking dish in an oven preheated to 350°F.

Calories per serving, one pepper, stuffed with ground turkey: 384. Percent of calories from fat 14%, protein 25%, carbohydrates 64%, 25 mg cholesterol.

Nutritional profile (% of RDA) per serving: Vitamin A - 106, Vitamin C - 371, Vitamin D - 41, Vitamin E - 45, Vitamin K - 52, Thiamine - 44, Riboflavin - 21, Niacin - 20, Vitamin B6 - 130, Folacin - 30, Vitamin B12 - 86, Pantothenic Acid - 28, Biotin - 9, Calcium - 9, Phosphorus - 38, Magnesium - 38, Potassium - 55, Sodium - 20, Iron - 35, Copper - 10, Manganese - 51, Zinc - 26, Selenium - 39, Chromium - 52.

✻ *Stuffed Squash*

Serves 8

Acorn squash is a native American gourd. It was originally called asquash by the Algonquin Indians. Acorn squash is sweeter than pumpkin and very high in vitamin A. Choose dark green gourds, free of cuts and bruises. This meal-in-one dish is fun to eat and decorative as an entree when served with a light soup or salad.

One pound ground turkey could be substituted for the tofu. Prepare it as in Stuffed Peppers.

<u>Rice</u>
31/2 cups chicken or vegetable broth
11/2 cups brown or basmati rice
2 medium size onions, chopped
1 tablespoon fresh ginger, peeled and grated
1 to 2 fresh chile peppers, seeded and minced
5 cloves garlic, minced
2 teaspoons coriander seeds
11/2 cup buckwheat groats
4 strips 3"x 1" kombu,
    soaked for 15 minutes and chopped

<u>Squash and Stuffing</u>
8 medium size acorn squashes
1 pound firm tofu, cubed
1/2 cup soy sauce
2 tablespoons fresh ginger, peeled and grated
1/4 cup mirin (Japanese rice wine) or dry sherry

1/4 cup water
2 cloves garlic, minced
1 cup green beans, chopped and lightly steamed
2 cups carrots, thinly sliced and lightly steamed
1 can (16 ounces) kidney beans, drained
2 tablespoons brewer's yeast

Preheat the oven to 350°F.

Place all 8 squashes in a large baking dish and bake for 30 minutes. When finished baking, remove the squashes from the oven and let them cool.

To prepare the rice, bring the broth to a boil in a 3-quart saucepan. Add all the other ingredients except the kombu and return to a boil. Lower the heat, cover, and simmer for 45 minutes, or until all liquids have been absorbed. Add the kombu halfway through the cooking time.

Meanwhile, mix together in a medium-size bowl the soy sauce, ginger, mirin, and water. Marinate the tofu for 30 minutes. Thoroughly drain the tofu and mix it with the rice and all the stuffing ingredients.

When the squashes are cool enough to handle, slice the top from each one and scoop out the seeds. Stuff each squash with the stuffing and top with its "lid." Bake 30 minutes.

There will be extra stuffing, which should be divided up and served alongside each squash.

To freeze: Any stuffed vegetable dish is easy to freeze, as the vegetable acts as a built-in container. Freezer baggies are more space saving than dishes for stuffed squash, as the squash itself is rather large. To thaw, place in the refrigerator overnight and reheat in the microwave or in a covered baking dish in an oven preheated to 350° F for 20 minutes.

Calories per serving of one squash with 1/8 total recipe of stuffing: 513. Percentage of calories from fat 9%, protein 19%, carbohydrate 72%, 0 mg cholesterol.

Nutritional profile (% of RDA) per serving: Vitamin A - 279, Vitamin C - 85, Vitamin D - 54, Vitamin E - 51, Vitamin K - 93, Thiamine - 136, Riboflavin - 46, Niacin - 42, Vitamin B6 - 73, Folacin - 116, Vitamin

B12 -60, Pantothenic Acid - 67, Biotin -14, Calcium - 25, Phosphorus -56, Magnesium - 94, Potassium - 116, Sodium - 101, Iron - 46, Copper - 42, Manganese - 83, Zinc - 30, Selenium - 55, Chromium - 76.

✳ Stuffed Potatoes and Creamed Cole Slaw

Serves 8

STUFFED POTATOES CAN BE GREAT PORTABLE MEALS, AND ARE BECOMING INCREASINGLY POPULAR. THIS DISH IS BOTH ECONOMICAL AND SIMPLE. TO QUALIFY NUTRITIONALLY AS A MEGAMEAL, THESE STUFFED POTATOES SHOULD BE SERVED WITH THE CREAMED COLE SLAW BELOW. THE CABBAGE AND EXTRA BUTTERMILK IN THE COLE SLAW ADD CALCIUM. THE COLE SLAW TAKES 5 MINUTES TO PREPARE WITH A FOOD PROCESSOR. WE SUGGEST THAT YOU PREPARE IT FRESH AS IT DOES NOT FREEZE WELL.

EQUALLY SATISFYING, ALTHOUGH NOT QUITE A MEGAMEAL, IS OUR VEGETARIAN VERSION BELOW.

<u>Stuffed Potatoes</u>
4 large baking potatoes
3 cans (8 ounces each) tuna, packed in water
1/2 pound fresh or frozen peas
1 cup minced celery, with leaves
1 medium-size red bell pepper, seeded and chopped fine
3 sheets (each 4" x 2") nori, shredded
1/2 cup minced dill pickle
2 cups buttermilk
2/3 cup nonfat dry milk
1/2 cup wheat germ
1 heaping tablespoon brewer's yeast
1/2 cup shredded low-fat or nonfat mozzarella cheese

Creamed Cole Slaw
1/4 head cabbage, shredded
4 carrots, grated
1/3 cup sunflower seeds
1/3 cup raisins
1/2 cup buttermilk
1 tablespoon balsamic or tarragon vinegar
1 teaspoon dried dill

Preheat the oven to 350°F. Line a large cookie sheet with foil.

Gently scrub the potatoes, leaving the skins intact. Bake for 45 minutes, or until a fork easily pierces the center. Remove from the oven, cut each potato in half, and let cool.

Drain the tuna well and flake into a large bowl. Mix in the peas, celery, red bell pepper, nori, and dill pickle. Toss the mixture with 1/4 cup buttermilk to moisten, then set aside.

Gently scoop out the potato meat. Leave the shells intact and set aside. Mash the potato meat with a fork or a potato masher, and blend in the nonfat dry milk, wheat germ, brewer's yeast, and approximately 1 to 1 1/2 cups buttermilk. Add more buttermilk as needed for moist yet not runny mashed potatoes.

Fill each potato shell three-fourths full with the mashed potato mixture. Divide the tuna salad equally among the potato halves and sprinkle the shredded mozzarella on top. Arrange on the foil-lined cookie sheet and bake 20 minutes.

Meanwhile, make the cole slaw. Mix together the cabbage, carrots, sunflower seeds, and raisins. In a shaker jar, mix the buttermilk, vinegar, and dill. Shake well. Use the dressing to moisten only; you will have more than you need. Use the extra dressing as a dip for the potatoes. (If you are keeping track of your calories, don't forget to count the calories in the dip you use.)

Turn the oven to broil. Brown the cheese topping on the potatoes for 3 minutes. Serve immediately with the cole slaw.

To freeze: Potatoes do not freeze as well as other vegetables, as they tend to dry out a little. But add nonfat yogurt to your reheated spud and you will never know the difference. Wrap each potato in freezer wax paper and store in freezer baggies. To thaw, place in the refrigerator overnight and reheat in the microwave or in a baking dish in an oven preheated to 350°F.

Calories per serving: 545. Percentage of calories from fat 29%, protein 55%, carbohydrates 20%, 19 mg cholesterol.

Nutritional profile (% of RDA) per serving: Vitamin A - 105, Vitamin C - 123, Vitamin D - 100, Vitamin E - 127, Vitamin K - 160, Thiamine - 155, Riboflavin - 70, Niacin - 87, Vitamin B6 - 211, Folacin - 119, Vitamin B12 - 197, Pantothenic Acid - 86, Biotin - 21, Calcium - 47, Phosphorus - 82, Magnesium - 69, Potassium - 114, Sodium - 60, Iron - 51, Copper - 60, Manganese - 62, Zinc - 42, Selenium - 251, Chromium - 116.

✳ *Vegetarian Stuffed Potatoes*

Replace the tuna in the recipe above with an additional 1 tablespoon nonfat dry milk and 1 teaspoon bran flakes (these contribute vitamin B12), stirring them into the mashed potato with the other ingredients. Fill the potato shells, top with the tuna-less salad and bake, without the mozzarella cheese. Remove from the oven after baking and top each with 1/4 cup plain nonfat yogurt mixed with 1 chopped hard-cooked egg and some minced fresh parsley or scallions.

Calories per serving: 464. Percentage of calories from fat 20%, protein 25%, carbohydrate 54%, 232 mg cholesterol.

✳ Pesto Quiche

Makes 2 quiches, serves 8

THIS IS A SIMPLE, QUICK RECIPE THAT I'VE MODIFIED FROM A QUICHE I TASTED AT THE GARLIC FESTIVAL IN GILROY, CALIFORNIA. WITH THE INCREASING POPULARITY OF PESTO, WE MAY SOON SEE A DISH SOMETHING LIKE THIS IN ITALIAN RESTAURANTS.

THIS IS A RECIPE FOR TWO QUICHES TO SERVE 8 PEOPLE — ONE SERVING IS ONE FOURTH OF ONE QUICHE.

NOTE THAT THE IRON IS SLIGHTLY UNDER THE 50-60 PERCENT OR MORE OF RECOMMENDED DAILY ALLOWANCES PROMISED IN A ONE-A-DAY MEGAMEAL. YOU MAY CONSIDER SERVING THEM WITH A SMALL PIECE OF LIVER SAUTEED WITH ONIONS, OR WITH FRESH OYSTERS, OR EVEN A SMALL BROILED STEAK.

YOU WILL NEED TWO 10-INCH QUICHE DISHES OR DEEP-DISH PIE PLATES. YOU COULD EVEN USE A LASAGNE BAKING PAN AND MAKE ONE LARGE QUICHE.

Crusts
2 cups water
8 ounces wild rice
2 medium-size sweet potatoes, peeled
1/2 cup wheat germ
1/4 cup whole-wheat flour
8 sheets (each 4" x 2") nori
1 tablespoon brewer's yeast

Filling
2 cups fresh basil
8 large cloves garlic
1/3 cup pumpkin seeds
1/3 cup grated Parmesan cheese
1/4 teaspoon black pepper
1/4 cup white wine
2 cups broccoli flowerets
2 cups low-fat or nonfat cottage cheese
1/2 cup buttermilk
6 egg whites, lightly beaten

4 scallions, white part only, chopped
1/2 cup chopped fresh parsley

Preheat the oven to 400°F.

To make the crusts, in a medium saucepan bring 2 cups water to a boil. Add the wild rice. Reduce the heat and simmer, covered, for 45 minutes, or until cooked thoroughly. Remove cover and fluff the rice with a fork.

In a food processor shred the sweet potatoes. Mix the raw sweet potato with the cooked wild rice, wheat germ, whole-wheat flour, nori, and brewer's yeast. Press over the bottom and sides of two 10"quiche or deep-dish pie plates. Bake for 20 to 30 minutes, or until the crust is crisp. After you remove the crusts from the oven, leave the oven on at 400°F.

For the fillings, place the basil and garlic in a food processor. Process briefly, until the basil is just chopped. Add the pumpkin seeds and chop for 1 minute. The seeds should be coarsely, not finely, ground. Add the cheese, pepper, and wine, and mix to blend only. The texture should be coarse rather than pureed. Set the pesto aside.

Steam the broccoli flowers for 5 minutes. You want to retain the bright green color of the broccoli, so do not overcook it: the vegetables should be crunchy, yet tender.

In a food processor blend the cottage cheese, buttermilk, and egg whites. Transfer to a large bowl and stir in the broccoli, scallions, parsley, and the pesto.

Fill the quiche crusts with the filling and bake for 20 minutes at 400°F, then reduce the heat to 350°F and continue to bake for another 15 to 20 minutes. The quiches should puff and turn golden. They are excellent served either hot or cold.

To freeze: Carefully slip each serving into a freezer baggie. This dish stacks economically in the freezer. To thaw, place in the refrigerator overnight and reheat in a baking dish in an oven preheated to 350°F for 15 minutes.

Calories per serving: 447. Percentage of calories from fat 12%, protein 20%, carbohydrates 67%, 13 mg cholesterol.

Nutritional profile (% of RDA) per serving: Vitamin A - 266, Vitamin C - 202, Vitamin D - 16, Vitamin E - 69, Vitamin K - 390, Thiamine - 65, Riboflavin - 45, Niacin - 21, Vitamin B6 - 63, Folacin - 55, Vitamin B12 - 41, Pantothenic Acid - 60, Biotin - 9, Calcium - 28, Phosphorus - 47, Magnesium - 33, Potassium - 52, Sodium - 49, Iron - 29, Copper - 14, Manganese - 40, Zinc - 20, Selenium - 29, Chromium - 56.

✳ Curry Quiche

Makes 2 quiches, serves 8

Prepare and bake the crusts as directed in the recipe for Pesto Quiche, above.

In a food processor combine 1/2 to 1 jalapeño chile, seeded and coarsely chopped, 1/3 cup toasted pumpkin seeds, 1/2 teaspoon each ground cumin and coriander, and 1/4 teaspoon ground turmeric. Process until the chile and pumpkin seeds are coarsely ground. Set aside.

Prepare the filling using the same ingredients as for the Pesto Quiche, but steam 2 cups sliced carrots instead of broccoli and use the jalapeño seasoning instead of the pesto. Fill and bake the quiche crusts as directed above.

Note: The nutritional figures will be approximately the same as the figures for the Pesto Quiche, but slightly lower because the Parmesan cheese is not used.

✳ Vegetable Quiche

Makes 2 quiches, serves 8

THERE IS A CHINESE ACCENT TO THIS TOFU-BASED QUICHE. THE SWEET POTATO CRUST AND THE CREAMY TOPPING MAKE IT A SCRUMPTIOUS CREATION. THE TOFU PUFFS UP AND BROWNS JUST LIKE A RICH CUSTARD, CROWNING THE FILLING AND CRISP, TOASTED CRUST. TOFU IS A WONDERFUL DAIRYLESS ALTER-NATIVE TO CHEESE, AND THIS QUICHE MAY TURN YOU INTO A TOFU LOVER. SERVE WITH A SIMPLE GREEN SALAD.

Crust
2 cups water
8 ounces wild rice
2 medium-size sweet potatoes, peeled
1/2 cup wheat germ
1/4 cup whole-wheat flour
8 sheets (each 4" x 2") nori
1 tablespoon brewer's yeast

Filling
3 medium-size eggplants, sliced into 1/4 inch rounds
Canola oil cooking spray
1/2 teaspoon sesame oil
2 tablespoons fresh ginger, peeled and minced
8 cloves garlic, minced
1 large onion, chopped
4 carrots, sliced into 1/4" pieces
4 ounces green beans, sliced into 1/4" pieces
1/4 cup water
8 shiitake mushrooms fresh or dried,
    soaked for 15 minutes, drained, and stemmed if dried,
    sliced into long thin strips
3/4 cup cooked garbanzo beans (chickpeas)
2 large fresh tomatoes, seeded and chopped
1 cup fresh or frozen peas, cooked

Seasoning sauce
3 tablespoons dry red wine
2 tablespoons rice vinegar
2 teaspoons low-sodium soy sauce
1/2 teaspoon sesame oil
1 teaspoon cornstarch mixed
    with 3 tablespoons water

Topping
2 10-ounce containers soft tofu
3 tablespoons lemon juice
1 tablespoon low-sodium soy sauce
1 teaspoon Chinese five-spice powder or dry mustard
1/2 teaspoon garlic powder
1/4 teaspoon black pepper

Garnish
1/4 cup chopped fresh parsley
Dash of paprika

Preheat the oven to 400° F.

Start the crust: In a medium-size saucepan, bring 2 cups water to a boil. Add the wild rice. Reduce the heat and simmer, covered, for 45 minutes, or until cooked through.

Meanwhile, arrange the eggplant rounds in a single layer on a cookie sheet sprayed with canola oil and bake for 10 minutes, until soft. This will probably take three shifts, depending on the size of your oven. When cool, cut the eggplant into 1/2 inch cubes. Set aside.

When the rice is cooked, uncover the pan and fluff with a fork. In a food processor shred the sweet potatoes. Mix the raw sweet potato with the cooked wild rice, wheat germ, flour, nori, and yeast. Press over the bottom and sides of two 10" quiche pans, deep dish pie plates or large baking dishes. Bake for 20 to 30 minutes or until the crust is crisp.

While the crust is baking, spray a large skillet with canola oil. Heat the skillet over low heat and add the sesame oil, ginger, and garlic. Stir-fry for a minute, then add the onion, carrots, green beans, and water. Cover and simmer for 15 minutes. Add the shiitake mushrooms, eggplant, garbanzo beans and tomatoes. Simmer for another 5 minutes.

In a small bowl beat all the ingredients for the seasoning sauce, except the cornstarch solution, to blend; then stir into the vegetables. Simmer 3 to 5 minutes. Most of the liquid should be absorbed. Stir in the peas. Slowly drizzle in the cornstarch solution, stirring constantly. Remove from the heat.

Combine all of the topping ingredients in a food processor and process till velvety smooth. The topping will be thick.

Remove the quiche crusts from the oven and turn the heat down to 350°F. Fill both crusts with vegetable filling and pour half of the topping over each. Sprinkle with paprika.

Bake for 30 minutes, or until set. Garnish with chopped fresh parsley before serving.

To freeze: Carefully slide each slice into freezerware plastic bags and freeze promptly. Thaw overnight in the refrigerator and reheat in a covered baking dish in an oven preheated to 350°F for 15 minutes, or microwave.

Calories per serving: 447. Percent of calories from fat 12%, protein 20%, carbohydrate 69%, 0 mg cholesterol.

Nutritional profile (% of RDA) per serving: Vitamin A - 181, Vitamin C - 57, Vitamin D - 27, Vitamin E - 60, Vitamin K - 78, Thiamine - 69, Riboflavin - 44, Niacin - 40, Vitamin B6 - 96, Folacin - 60, Vitamin B12 - 53, Pantothenic Acid - 43, Biotin - 7, Calcium - 18, Phosphorus - 45, Magnesium - 69, Potassium - 94, Sodium - 10, Iron - 51, Copper - 24, Manganese - 62, Zinc - 24, Selenium - 25, Chromium - 49.

✳ Salmon Quiche

Makes 2 quiches, serves 8

THIS IS HALFWAY BETWEEN A QUICHE AND A FRITTATA. SERVE WITH MIXED GREENS WITH POPPY SEED DRESSING.

Crust
2 medium-size sweet potatoes
2 cups cooked brown rice
1/3 cup wheat germ
1 sheet (4" x 2") nori, cut up
1 tablespoon brewer's yeast

Filling
4 large stalks broccoli, flowerets only
4 large dried shiitake mushrooms, soaked 15 minutes,
drained, stemmed and sliced into long, thin strips
Olive oil cooking spray
1 1/2 cups cooked white beans
2 medium-size red bell peppers, seeded and chopped fine
1 large can or jar artichoke hearts
    packed in water, drained, halved

Topping
2 cups low-fat or nonfat cottage cheese
1 can (8 ounces) salmon
6 egg whites, lightly beaten
1 teaspoon dried marjoram
1/2 teaspoon minced fresh dill

Preheat the oven to 350°F.

In a food processor shred the sweet potatoes. Mix with the brown rice, wheat germ, nori, and yeast and press into two 9-inch quiche pans or pie plates. Bake for 20 to 30 minutes, or until the crust is crisp. When you remove the crusts from the oven, leave the oven on at 350°F.

Meanwhile, steam the broccoli. Lightly sauté the shiitake mushrooms in a small skillet sprayed with olive oil. Mix the beans with the bell peppers and set aside.

Evenly divide the artichoke hearts between the two quiche crusts and arrange them in a circle on the outer edges. Spoon half of the bean and pepper mix in a ring inside each circle of artichokes, then add a ring of half of the broccoli. Fill the center of each with the shiitake mushrooms.

For topping, whip the cottage cheese in a food processor for 1 minute, or until velvety smooth. Add the salmon and puree for 1 minute. Add all remaining ingredients and blend for another 30 seconds. Pour half of the topping over each quiche and bake for 30 minutes. Allow to cool for 10 minutes before slicing.

To freeze: Place each serving of quiche into freezer baggies. Especially with fish, once cooked, freeze promptly. To thaw, place overnight in the refrigerator. Reheat in a covered baking dish in an oven preheated to 350° F for 15 minutes, or microwave.

Calories per serving: 416. Percent of calories from fat 15%, protein 28%, carbohydrates 57%, 15 mg cholesterol.

Nutritional profile (% of RDA) per serving: Vitamin A - 83, Vitamin C - 129, Vitamin D - 53, Vitamin E - 82, Vitamin K - 199, Thiamine - 102, Riboflavin - 43, Niacin - 46, Vitamin B6 - 75, Folacin - 83, Vitamin B12 - 128, Pantothenic Acid - 57, Biotin - 17, Calcium - 19, Phosphorus - 52, Magnesium - 42, Potassium - 75, Sodium - 25, Iron - 36, Copper - 25, Manganese - 64, Zinc - 75, Selenium - 50, Chromium - 47.

✳ *Mussels Florentine*

Serves 4

MUSSELS ARE MAKING A COMEBACK IN CALIFORNIA. THEY ARE HIGH IN PROTEIN, CALCIUM, AND IRON, LOW IN FAT, AND ECONOMICAL. THEY HAVE A RICHER TASTE THAN EITHER OYSTERS OR CLAMS, AND ARE EASY TO PREPARE.

MAKE SURE MUSSELS ARE ALIVE WHEN YOU BEGIN COOKING. SHELLS YOU CAN WIGGLE BACK AND FORTH ARE SUSPECT, AND DISCARD ANY MUSSELS THAT SMELL STRANGE. THEY SHOULD SMELL SALTY, LIKE THE SEA. LIVE MUSSELS WILL OPEN DURING COOKING. DISCARD ANY THAT REMAIN CLOSED.

4 pounds mussels (1 pound per person,
   weight with shell)
2 cups dry white wine
1 cup clam juice
1/4 cup lemon juice
4 cloves garlic, minced
10 scallions, whites only, chopped
1 1/2 tablespoon fresh dill

**1 pound fresh spinach,cleaned and chopped
  or 1 package (10 ounces) frozen spinach,
  prepared according to package directions
12 ounces whole-wheat fettuccine noodles
4 fresh plum tomatoes, chopped
1 sheet (6" x 3") nori, cut into long, thin strips
Black pepper to taste
1/4 cup chopped fresh parsley**

To prepare the mussels, scrub the shells. Just prior to cooking, pull off the "beards." We advise against pulling the beards off far ahead of cooking because the stress on the mussel will usually kill it within a few hours, and you want the mussels to be fresh up until the moment you cook them. Store mussels in a colander or a paper bag, never plastic, so they can breathe.

In a large stockpot bring the wine, clam and lemon juices, garlic, scallions, and dill to a boil over high heat. Add the mussels. Cover and steam for 5 to 6 minutes only. Mussels cook faster than any other shellfish and will become tough if overdone. Drain the mussels, reserving and straining the broth. When cool, remove the mussels from the shell and return to the broth.

Steam the spinach. Cook the noodles according to the package instructions and drain.

Add the noodles, tomatoes, nori, and spinach to the broth and mussels. Heat gently. Add the black pepper to taste and stir in the parsley to serve.

To freeze: This dish does freeze well, although we do recommend that you chop a fresh tomato to serve either on the side or mix in with the noodles. Divide the noodles into equal portions and ladle into freezer baggies. To thaw, leave in the refrigerator overnight and reheat in a double boiler or in the microwave.

Calories per serving: 419. Percent of calories from fat 4%, protein 28%, carbohydrates 67%, 50 mg cholesterol.

Nutritional profile (% of RDA) per serving: Vitamin A - 116, Vitamin C - 98, Vitamin D - 27, Vitamin E - 34, Vitamin K - 86, Thiamine - 51, Riboflavin - 30, Niacin - 31, Vitamin B6 - 97, Folacin -

49, Vitamin B12 - 54, Pantothenic Acid - 35, Biotin - 15, Calcium - 17,
Phosphorus - 50, Magnesium - 55, Potassium - 65, Sodium - 36, Iron
- 55, Copper - 23, Manganese - 20, Zinc - 25, Selenium - 897,
Chromium - 57.

✳ Chow Mein

Serves 4

WE STRONGLY SUGGEST THAT YOU DOUBLE THIS RECIPE FOR TWO REA-
SONS: 1) THERE IS A LOT OF CHOPPING AND MINCING, AND IT IS
MORE SATISFYING TO PREPARE A DOUBLED RECIPE ONCE THAN TO PREPARE A
SINGLE RECIPE TWICE; AND 2) THIS DISH FREEZES EXTREMELY WELL. IT IS
ONE OF OUR FAVORITE MEALS!
    THE NOODLES ARE BAKED INSTEAD OF FRIED. THEY ARE CRISPER AND
LIGHTER THAN THEIR TRADITIONAL CHINESE PAN-FRIED NOODLE COUSINS. USE
THE BAKED NOODLES WITH ANY ORIENTAL SAUCE, IN OTHER STIR-FRY DISHES,
FOR A CRUNCHY SURPRISE OR PLAIN AS A SNACK.

    Canola oil cooking spray
    1 large eggplant, peeled
        and sliced into 1/4" rounds
    Salt
    2 teaspoons dry red wine
    2 teaspoons dark soy sauce
    1/2 cup chicken or vegetable stock
    2 teaspoons Chinese brown vinegar
        or regular rice vinegar
    1/2 teaspoon sesame oil
    1 container (10 ounces) firm tofu,
        drained and cut into 1-inch cubes
    1 tablespoon peeled and minced ginger
    2 cloves garlic, minced
    2 scallions, whites only, minced
    3 strips (each 3" x 1") kombu,
        soaked for 10 minutes and chopped

1 1/2 large red bell peppers, roasted (page 105)
1 1/2 large green bell peppers, roasted
3 cups washed and chopped fresh spinach
6 medium-size fresh shiitake mushrooms,
    sliced into thin strips
Tabasco to taste
2 tablespoons wheat germ
1 teaspoon cornstarch mixed with with
3 tablespoons chicken or vegetable broth or water
Chow Mein Noodles (recipe below)

Preheat the oven to 350°F. Spray a nonstick cookie sheet with canola oil.

To remove bitter juices from the eggplant, sprinkle salt onto both sides of the rounds, pile into a bowl, and let sit for 10 minutes.

Meanwhile, in a medium-size bowl beat the red wine, dark soy sauce, broth, vinegar, and 1/2 teaspoon of the sesame oil to blend. Add the tofu and toss well, then set aside to marinate.

Rinse the salt off each eggplant round and pat dry. Lay the rounds on the prepared cookie sheet and bake for 15 minutes, or until tender; do not overcook. When cool enough to handle, slice into 3" x 1" strips.

Coat a large nonstick skillet lightly with the remaining 1/2 teaspoon sesame oil. Heat until hazy and stir-fry the ginger, garlic, and scallions quickly, about 10 seconds. Stir in the eggplant, kombu, roasted pepper strips, spinach, mushrooms, tofu and its marinade, and Tabasco to taste. Stir-fry over low heat for 5 minutes. Stir in the wheat germ. Stirring constantly, drizzle the cornstarch mixture over the vegetables. Adding more liquid as necessary, cook until the sauce thickens. Gently stir in the noodles. Serve hot!

To Freeze: Noodle dishes are easy to freeze. Store equal portions in either freezerware dishes or baggies. To thaw, place in your refrigerator overnight. Reheat in the microwave, in a double boiler, or in a casserole dish in an oven preheated to 350°F for 15 minutes.

Chow Mein Noodles
Canola oil cooking spray
8 ounces whole-wheat fettuccini noodles
1 1/2 tablespoons chicken or vegetable broth

1 teaspoon low-sodium soy sauce
1/2 teaspoon sesame oil
1/4 teaspoon white pepper

Preheat the oven to 350°F. Spray an 8" square baking pan with canola oil.

Prepare the noodles according to package instructions. Meanwhile, in a large bowl beat the broth, soy sauce, sesame oil, and pepper to blend.

Drain the noodles well, then add to the mixture in the bowl and toss to mix. Spread the noodles in the prepared pan and bake for 10 minutes. Turn the noodles and bake on the other side for 5 minutes. Turn the oven to broil and broil the noodles for 3 minutes, or until crispy.

Break the cooked noodles gently into thick pieces.

Calories per serving (with noodles): 605. Percentage of calories from fat 10%, protein 19%, carbohydrates 70%, 0 mg cholesterol.

Nutritional profile (% of RDA) per serving: Vitamin A - 134, Vitamin C - 272, Vitamin D - 81, Vitamin E - 51, Vitamin K - 105, Thiamine - 71, Riboflavin - 48, Niacin - 55, Vitamin B6 - 71, Folacin - 59, Vitamin B12 - 90, Pantothenic Acid - 41, Biotin - 13, Calcium - 25, Phosphorus - 61, Magnesium - 99, Potassium - 167, Sodium - 26, Iron - 59, Copper - 13, Manganese - 48, Zinc - 24, Selenium - 142, Chromium - 66.

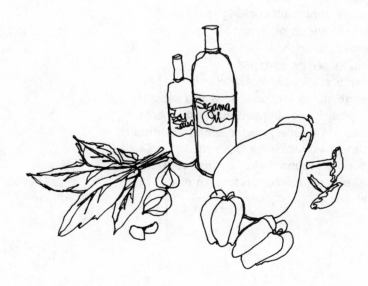

☀ *Manicotti*

Serves 8

Be sure to try this recipe. Its sweet potato-cheese filling, as surprising as that may sound, makes this manicotti incredibly rich. I've omitted the mozzarella, but there are low-fat and nonfat varieties that could be added to this recipe. The sauce is quite chunky with carrots, shiitake mushrooms, and freshly steamed broccoli added at the last minute. The manicotti makes an extravagantly scrumptious meal if you can find the noodles and have the time to stuff each one. If not, lasagne noodles work just as well, and instructions are given below for how to layer a lasagne. As for broccoli, ounce per ounce, the flowerets contain nearly eight times as much of the vitamin A compound beta-carotene as the stalks. Stalks still provide vitamins C and B, calcium, and fiber in addition to vitamin A. Broccoli is indeed a superfood!

<u>Stuffing</u>
1 large sweet potato, cooked
    (either baked or boiled) and peeled
8 ounces low-fat or nonfat ricotta cheese
3 scallions, whites only, chopped
2 tablespoons fresh parsley, chopped

<u>Sauce</u>
Olive or canola oil cooking spray
5 cloves garlic, minced
1 onion, chopped
3 stalks celery, chopped
3 carrots, sliced into 1/4"rounds
3 large stalks broccoli, flowerets separated, stalks
    peeled and chopped into 1/4" pieces
1 can (24 ounces) peeled tomatoes, drained
1 can (24 ounces) tomato sauce
8 ounces ground turkey or firm tofu, minced
Half of a six-ounce can tomato paste
4 sheets (8" x 5") nori

1 tablespoons low-sodium soy sauce
8 ounces fresh shiitake mushrooms, chopped
2 tablespoons wheat germ
1 ounce bran flakes
2 tablespoons chopped fresh oregano or 2 teaspoons dried
2 tablespoons chopped fresh basil or 2 teaspoons dried
Salt and black pepper to taste
1 1/2 pounds manicotti or lasagne noodles
1/4 cup grated Parmesan cheese

Preheat the oven to 350°F.

Spray a large nonstick skillet with olive oil. Over medium heat, stir 3 cloves of the garlic until it begins to brown. Add the onion, celery, carrots and broccoli stalks. Add 1/4 cup peeled tomatoes. Cook over medium heat until the vegetables are barely soft. Remove from the heat and save in a large pot.

Return the skillet to the stove and brown the remaining 2 cloves garlic. Reduce the heat and add the turkey. Stir while the turkey browns, breaking up the clumps. Mix the turkey in with the vegetables, along with the remaining tomatoes, tomato sauce, tomato paste, and nori.

Spray the skillet with more oil and return to the heat. Add the soy sauce and shiitake mushrooms and stir-fry until the mushrooms are soft and chewy. They may even dry-fry for a short time. Add to the vegetable and turkey sauce and heat over medium heat until barely boiling.

Meanwhile, in a separate pot, steam the broccoli flowerets.

Add the wheat germ, bran flakes, herbs, and salt and pepper to the sauce. Cook noodles over a low flame for 30 minutes while you prepare the stuffing and noodles.

Mash the sweet potato in a food processor. Add the ricotta cheese and blend until velvety smooth. Mix in the scallions and parsley. Set the stuffing aside.

Cook noodles according to package directions. Drain, then rinse under cold water.

Spray a large baking pan with canola oil. Spread a large spoonful of sauce over the bottom of the pan. If you are using manicotti noodles, stuff each noodle with the filling and arrange in the baking pan.

Stir the broccoli flowerets into the sauce and pour the sauce over all. If you are using lasagne noodles, layer half of the noodles, all of the filling, then the remaining noodles, and spread the sauce with the broccoli evenly over all. Sprinkle with Parmesan cheese and bake for 30 minutes.

To freeze: Whether you make the lasagne or the manicotti, simply divide into equal portions and store in freezer baggies. Thaw overnight in the refrigerator and reheat in the microwave or place in an uncovered baking dish in an oven preheated to 350°F for 20 minutes.

Calories per serving (with turkey): 623. Percent of calories from fat 13%, protein 20%, carbohydrates 66%, 35 mg cholesterol.

Nutritional profile (% of RDA) per serving: Vitamin A - 220, Vitamin C - 328, Vitamin D - 30, Vitamin E - 46, Vitamin K - 425, Thiamine - 69, Riboflavin - 53, Niacin - 53, Vitamin B6 - 121, Folacin - 61, Vitamin B12 - 64, Pantothenic Acid - 83, Biotin - 16, Calcium - 28, Phosphorus - 61, Magnesium - 59, Potassium - 137, Sodium - 24, Iron - 58, Copper - 17, Manganese - 28, Zinc - 81, Selenium - 105, Chromium - 95.

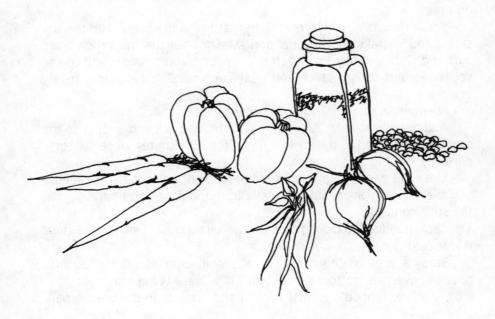

✳ *Lasagne*

Serves 8

SOMETIMES CALLED SOUTHWEST LASAGNE, THIS LASAGNE'S BLACK BEAN CHILE SAUCE AND KALE MAKE FOR A VERY HEARTY DISH. SERVE WITH A GREEN SALAD. TRADITIONAL SOUTHWEST CHILI ALMOST ALWAYS INCLUDES STEAK. YOU MAY CHOOSE TO OMIT THE EGGS AND BLEND OPTIONAL STEAK IN WITH THE BEAN MIX.

COMPARING EQUAL AMOUNTS OF STEAK TO EGGS IS ENLIGHTENING. ONE WHOLE EGG HAS 79 CALORIES AND WEIGHS 50 GRAMS, WHICH IS A LITTLE UNDER 2 OUNCES. AN EQUAL SERVING OF FLANK STEAK, SLIGHTLY UNDER 2 OUNCES, HAS 80 CALORIES. THE FAT CONTENT IN THE EGG IS ALMOST DOUBLE THE STEAK, BUT THE NUTRITIONAL VALUE IS SUBSTANTIALLY HIGHER. YOU GET MUCH MORE FOR YOUR 80 CALORIES FROM THE EGG. IN FACT, WITH THE EXCEPTION OF NIACIN, B6, AND PERHAPS IRON, THE EGG WINS HANDS DOWN OVER THE STEAK. EVEN THE VITAMIN B12 IN ONE WHOLE EGG WOULD FEED YOU FOR THE DAY. IF YOU ARE WATCHING YOUR CHOLESTEROL, THEN THIS IS A MOOT POINT (ONE EGG HAS 274 MG, WHILE THE FLANK STEAK HAS ONLY 27). THE EGG IS A NUTRIENT-RICH FOOD WHEN YOU SURROUND IT WITH PLENTY OF VEGETABLES AND GRAINS TO COUNTER THE FAT CONTENT. I USE EGG WHITES ALMOST DAILY (NO CHOLESTEROL) AND WHOLE EGGS A FEW TIMES A WEEK.

2 pounds kale
Olive oil cooking spray
1/3 pound flank steak,
      fat trimmed, cubed (optional)
A1 sauce, to taste
3 cups cooked black beans
3 strips (each 3" x 1") kombu,
      soaked for 10 minutes and chopped
1 tablespoon brewer's yeast
2/3 cup cooked corn
1/2 cup chopped onion
1 large red bell pepper, seeded and diced
1 large fresh tomato, chopped
1 1/2 cups low-fat or nonfat cottage cheese
1 cup low-fat or nonfat yogurt

3 eggs
1/4 cup wheat germ
1/3 cup bran flakes
1 pound whole-wheat lasagne noodles
2/3 of a 6-ounce can tomato paste
1 cup water
1/2 teaspoon dried oregano
1 teaspoon ground cumin
2 cloves garlic, minced
2 serrano chiles, seeded and minced
1/4 cup chopped fresh cilantro

Preheat oven to 350°F.

Steam the kale for 10 minutes, or until the leaves are tender. Set aside.

If you are adding steak, spray a medium-size skillet with olive oil. Sear the steak over a medium flame for 2 minutes. Reduce the heat, add a little water, some A1 sauce, and cover. Simmer the steak cubes for 5 minutes.

Mix the black beans, kombu, (steak), and yeast together in a large bowl. In a separate bowl mix together the corn, onion, red pepper, and tomato and set aside. In a third bowl mix the cheese, yogurt, eggs, wheat germ, and bran flakes.

Fill a large pot two thirds full of water and bring to a boil. Cook the noodles for 12 to 15 minutes. Drain, then rinse under cold water, separating each noodle.

Make a sauce by placing a small saucepan over medium heat and adding 1 cup water to the tomato paste. Stir thoroughly, then add the oregano, cumin, garlic, and chiles. Simmer over low heat for 20 minutes.

This is a dish of many layers. Line the bottom of a lasagne pan with the steamed kale. Spread a fine layer of bean mixture over the kale. Lightly spread with one third of the tomato sauce mixture. Follow this with a layer of noodles, a layer of vegetables, and a layer of cheese mixture. Sprinkle on all the cilantro. Repeat with the remainder of the beans (and steak), half of the remaining tomato sauce, half the remaining noodles, the remaining vegetable mixture, all of the cheese mixture and the final layer of noodles. Pour the rest of the tomato sauce over the top of the lasagne. Bake the lasagne for 45 minutes, and allow to cool for 10.

   To freeze: This freezes very well. Store generous slices in freezer-ware or baggies. Thaw overnight in the refrigerator and reheat in the microwave or place uncovered in a baking dish in an oven preheated to 350°F for 20 minutes.

Calories per serving (without meat): 608. Percent of calories from fat 10%, protein 57%, carbohydrates 29%, 57 mg cholesterol.

Nutritional profile (% of RDA) per serving: Vitamin A - 250, Vitamin C - 345, Vitamin D - 100, Vitamin E - 104, Vitamin K - 58, Thiamine - 133, Riboflavin - 64, Niacin - 58, Vitamin B6 - 100, Folacin - 108, Vitamin B12 - 152, Pantothenic Acid - 78, Biotin - 15, Calcium - 38, Phosphorus - 69, Magnesium - 75, Potassium - 122, Sodium - 59, Iron - 60, Copper - 31, Manganese - 50, Zinc - 38, Selenium - 95, Chromium - 56.

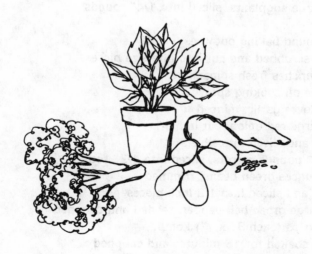

✳ *Moussaka*

Serves 8

IN BROWSING THROUGH THIS BOOK, YOU WILL FIND A NUMBER OF DIFFER-
ENT TOPPING PREPARATIONS IN THE RECIPES FOR QUICHES, VEGETABLE PÂTÉ
AND VEGETABLE MOUSSAKA. THESE TOPPINGS ARE BASICALLY INTERCHANGE-
ABLE. SOME ARE TOFU BASED, SOME POTATO BASED, AND ONE IS MAKE WITH
EVAPORATED SKIM MILK. THIS ONE IS YOGURT BASED, AND USES EGG WHITES
TO SET INTO A CUSTARDLIKE SAUCE.

A NOTE ABOUT THE LAMB. IT IS IMPORTANT TO GET THE LOIN OF THE
LAMB, IF POSSIBLE, BECAUSE IT IS THE LEANEST OF LAMB CUTS. IF YOU GET
IT FROM A BUTCHER, HE WILL GRIND IT FOR YOU. IF YOU HAVE YOUR OWN MEAT
GRINDER, FINE. IF THE ONLY THING AVAILABLE TO YOU IS PLAIN "GROUND
LAMB" FROM YOUR SUPERMARKET, THEN BE SURE TO DRAIN OFF THE FAT AS
YOU COOK IT, BECAUSE PLAIN GROUND LAMB IS VERY FATTY.

SERVE THIS WITH ORANGE VEGETABLE SOUP AND A MIXED GREEN SALAD.

<u>Moussaka</u>
2 large eggplants, sliced into 1/4" rounds
Salt
1 pound baking potatoes,
    scrubbed and cut into bite-size pieces
2 bunches fresh spinach
Olive oil cooking spray
8 cloves garlic, minced
1 large red onion, cut in half
    and sliced into slivers
11/2 pounds carrots, sliced into 1/2" rounds
8 ounces green beans, trimmed
    and sliced into 1/2-inch pieces
1 large green bell pepper, seeded and chopped
3 strips (each 3" x 1") kombu,
    soaked for 15 minutes and chopped
1 pound lamb loin, ground
1 teaspoon black pepper
Pinch of dried rosemary
2 tablespoons brewer's yeast

3 tablespoons paprika
1/2 cup bran flakes
1/4 cup whole-wheat flour

Topping
2 cups low-fat or nonfat yogurt
1/2 cup wheat germ
6 egg whites, at room temperature
Freshly grated nutmeg to taste

Preheat oven to 350°F.

Slice eggplant into 1/4" rounds. Sprinkle liberally with salt, pile into a large bowl and let them "sweat" out their bitter juices for 10 minutes. Rinse them thoroughly, pat dry, and set aside.

In a medium saucepan, boil the potatoes in water to cover for 5 minutes. Drain and set aside. Wash the spinach, and steam briefly, 5 minutes at most; the spinach should retain its bright green color. Set aside.

Spray a large nonstick skillet with olive oil and brown the garlic over low heat. Add a little water and cook the onion, carrots, green beans, bell pepper, and kombu until just tender. Add the lamb, black pepper, and rosemary. Cook over medium heat 5 to 10 minutes, stirring often, until the meat is just cooked. Add the cooked potatoes. Stir in the yeast and paprika.

Combine the bran flakes and flour. Dip the eggplant rounds in this mixture, coating evenly on all sides.

Cover the bottom of a 13" x 7" baking pan with the spinach. Alternate layers of eggplant with the vegetable/lamb mixture, beginning with the eggplant and ending with the lamb.

To make the topping, whip the yogurt and wheat germ together in a blender until creamy and light. Using an electric mixer or whisk, beat the egg whites until stiff peaks form. Fold the egg whites into the yogurt mixture. Spoon over the moussaka. Top with fresh nutmeg.

Bake for 20 minutes. Remove briefly, and set the oven to broil. Broil the moussaka for 3 to 5 minutes, until the topping puffs up golden, like a meringue.

To freeze: Freezerware dishes or freezer baggies serve equally well for freezing this dish. Thaw overnight in the refrigerator and reheat in the microwave or in a baking dish in an oven preheated to 350°F for 15 minutes.

Calories per serving: 525. Percent of calories from fat 22%, protein 38%, carbohydrates 40%, 47 mg cholesterol.

Nutritional profile (% of RDA) per serving: Vitamin A - 287, Vitamin C - 174, Vitamin D - 114, Vitamin E - 90, Vitamin K - 230, Thiamine - 182, Riboflavin - 92, Niacin - 68, Vitamin B6 - 119, Folacin - 174, Vitamin B12 - 220, Pantothenic Acid - 96, Biotin - 26, Calcium - 48, Phosphorus - 80, Magnesium - 103, Potassium - 166, Sodium - 62, Iron - 59, Copper - 51, Manganese - 81, Zinc - 51, Selenium - 79, Chromium - 102.

❋ *Vegetable Moussaka*

Serves 6

THIS IS AN ADAPTATION OF THE TRADITIONAL GREEK FAVORITE. WE OUR-SELVES USE MUCH MORE SLIVERED GARLIC THAN THE 8 CLOVES SUGGESTED HERE, AND WE SPRINKLE THE GARLIC BETWEEN EVERY LAYER, BUT WE WILL LEAVE THAT TO YOUR PALATE!

BESIDES BEING USED AS A CONDIMENT, GARLIC HAS LONG BEEN KNOWN TO HAVE MEDICINAL USES. THOUGH SOME OF THE CLAIMS FOR ITS MEDICINAL EFFECTS ARE MYTHS, SOME ARE TRUE. IT DOES LOWER CERTAIN RISK FACTORS FOR ARTERIOSCLEROTIC HEART DISEASE, AND IT DEPRESSES THE SYNTHESIS OF CHOLESTEROL FROM GLYCEROL IN THE LIVER. ALSO, THE ORGANOSULFUR COM-POUNDS IN GARLIC SHOW SOME ANTI-CANCER ACTIVITY, AND STUDIES SUGGEST THAT IT DOES INDEED OFFER SOME CANCER PROTECTION.

Moussaka
31/2 cups water
1/4 cup dried soybeans, soaked overnight and drained
1 cup barley
2 large eggplants, sliced into 1/4 inch rounds
Salt
Canola oil cooking spray

6 carrots, sliced into 1/4" rounds
8 ounces green beans, trimmed
    and sliced into 1/2" pieces
8 ounces Swiss chard or beet greens
1/2 cup sunflower seeds
1/2 cup pumpkin seeds
1/4 cup wheat germ
1 tablespoon brewer's yeast
8 cloves garlic (or more), minced
1 teaspoon chopped fresh basil
1 teaspoon dried marjoram
2 large onions, sliced into 1/4" rounds
3 large fresh tomatoes, sliced into 1/4" rounds
2 sheets nori (4" x 2"), cut or coarsely chopped

Béchamel Sauce
1 can (12 ounces) evaporated skim milk
1/2 cup vegetable broth
1/4 cup oat (or whole-wheat) flour
1/4 cup nonfat dry milk
1/4 teaspoon white pepper
1/4 teaspoon nutmeg
Paprika to taste

Preheat the oven to 450°F.

In a large kettle or pot heat 3 1/2 cups of water to boiling. Add the soybeans and barley, reduce the heat, and simmer, covered, for 1 hour. The soybeans should be slightly crunchy, and the barley cooked. Set aside.

Slice the eggplants into 1/4" rounds. Drizzle each side with salt, pile into a large bowl and let the eggplant "sweat" for 10 minutes. Rinse the salt off the eggplant rounds and pat dry. Spray two cookie sheets with canola oil, and arrange eggplant rounds in one layer each on sheet. Bake one sheet on each oven shelf for 10 minutes. Remove from oven and set aside, lowering the oven temperature to 350°F.

Steam carrots and green beans for 7 minutes, merely to tenderize them a little, they will finish cooking in the oven. Steam the chard for 5 minutes, then drain, pressing out as much of the cooking juices as possible. Set aside.

Chop the sunflower and pumpkin seeds briefly in a food processor. Keep them chunky; do not overgrind into a paste. Mix the seeds with the cooked barley and soybeans. Stir in the wheat germ and yeast and set aside.

Mix the minced garlic in a separate dish with the basil and marjoram.

To make the béchamel sauce, combine the evaporated milk with the broth in a medium saucepan. Sift in the oat flour, a little at a time, using a wire whisk to blend. Add the nonfat dry milk, stirring constantly. Heat over a low flame, whisking constantly for 5 minutes, or until it thickens. Stir in the pepper and nutmeg.

Line two 8"x 8" baking dishes with the chard, followed by one third of the eggplant. Next add all of the carrots and green beans. Sprinkle half of the garlic-herb seasoning over the vegetables. Spread the barley-bean layer over the carrots. Layer in the sliced onions, and next the tomatoes. Sprinkle on another layer of garlic herbs along with the nori. Top the dish with a final layer of eggplant. Pour the béchamel sauce over the moussaka and sprinkle with paprika.

Bake for 1 hour at 350°F.

Serve with the following Hummus Sauce.

Hummus Sauce
Makes about 1 cup
1/2 cup cooked garbanzo beans (chickpeas)
2 cloves garlic, coarsely chopped
1/2 cup vegetable broth
1 tablespoon onion powder
2 tablespoons chopped fresh parsley

Puree all the ingredients except the parsley in a food processor. Heat the sauce in a small saucepan over low heat. Just prior to serving, stir in the parsley.

To freeze: Follow the directions for freezing in the previous recipe.

Calories per serving (with 2 tablespoons Hummus Sauce): 569. Percent of calories from fat 25%, protein 35%, carbohydrates 65%, 4 mg cholesterol.

Nutritional profile (% of RDA) per serving (with 2 tablespoons of Hummus Sauce): Vitamin A - 283, Vitamin C - 100, Vitamin D - 25, Vitamin E - 107, Vitamin K - 155, Thiamine - 92, Riboflavin - 75, Niacin - 48, Vitamin B6 - 94, Folacin - 91, Vitamin B12 - 54, Pantothenic Acid - 85, Biotin - 28, Calcium - 45, Phosphorus - 73, Magnesium - 63, Potassium - 156, Sodium - 33, Iron - 61, Copper - 61, Manganese - 187, Zinc - 33, Selenium - 80, Chromium - 77.

✳*Vegetable Pâté with Velvet Sauce*

Serves 8

THIS MEAT-FREE PÂTÉ IS TEN TIMES MORE NUTRITIOUS THAN A CLASSIC PÂTÉ OR MEAT LOAF. THE BEANS GIVE IT A HEARTY CHARACTER, WHILE THE VELVET SAUCE MELTS ON YOUR TONGUE. IT IS WONDERFUL SERVED HOT OR COLD, AND IS GREAT FOR SANDWICHES.

> 5 cups vegetable broth
> 1 cup soybeans, soaked overnight
> 1 piece (3" x 3") kombu,
>   soaked for 15 minutes, drained and chopped
> 2 cups lentils
> 8 ounces kale
> 2 cups unsweetened all-bran cereal
> 2/3 cup wheat germ
> 2/3 cup rolled oats
> 6 egg whites
> 1 can (12 ounces) evaporated skim milk
> 8 medium-size carrots, grated
> 1 large onion, chopped
> 1 tablespoon Worcestershire sauce
> 1 tablespoon dill
> 1 teaspoon black pepper
> Canola oil cooking spray

Preheat the oven to 350°F.

Fill a large saucepan with the vegetable broth and bring to a boil. Add the soybeans and cook, covered, over low heat for 20 minutes. Add the kombu and lentils, and continue to cook for another 15 minutes. Add the kale and cook for a final 15 minutes. Check the beans and cook a little longer if necessary. The soybeans should be a little crunchy. Remove from the heat and set aside.

In a food processor, blend the bran cereal into a bread crumb consistency, and mix with the wheat germ and rolled oats. In a large bowl lightly whip the egg whites with a fork. Add the bran mixture, beans, milk, carrots, onion, Worcestershire, dill, and pepper; mix together well.

Spray a decorative baking mold or 9" x 12" baking pan with canola oil. Firmly press the pâté mixture into place. It will be a good 3 inches high. Bake for 35 to 45 minutes, until firm but not dry.

If you are eating the pâté hot from the oven, serve with two heaping tablespoons warm Velvet Sauce and a simple cooked grain. If you are eating it chilled, serve with chilled Velvet Sauce and a smooth-textured, soft whole-wheat bread.

Velvet Sauce
Makes about 2 cups.
1/4 cup sesame tahini
1/4 cup water
2 cloves garlic, coarsely chopped
2 tablespoons Chinese brown rice vinegar
    or regular rice vinegar
1 tablespoon low-sodium soy sauce
1 tablespoon lemon juice
1 container (10 ounces) soft tofu, drained
Salt and white pepper to taste

In a blender or food processor, combine the tahini, water, garlic, vinegar, soy sauce, and lemon juice and process until smooth. Add the soft tofu, and blend briefly. Transfer the mixture to a small saucepan and add salt and white pepper to taste. Heat briefly and serve. This Velvet Sauce is delicious chilled as well. Serve on chilled plates.

To freeze: This pâté can be served hot or cold, but should be frozen in appropriate single servings in freezer baggies. It thaws more quickly than the other recipes; in three hours on the kitchen counter. Do not leave it out without refrigeration for longer than that. Reheat in the microwave or wrap in aluminum foil and bake in a preheated 350°F oven for 12 minutes.

Calories per serving (with 2 tablespoons Velvet Sauce): 492. Percent of calories from fat 14%, protein 25%, carbohydrate 60%, 1 mg cholesterol.

Nutritional profile (% of RDA) per serving (with 2 tablespoons of Velvet Sauce): Vitamin A - 235, Vitamin C - 115, Vitamin D - 27, Vitamin E - 120, Vitamin K - 210, Thiamine - 104, Riboflavin - 64, Niacin - 48, Vitamin B6 - 85, Folacin - 40, Vitamin B12 - 94, Pantothenic Acid - 65, Biotin - 24, Calcium - 27, Phosphorus - 69, Magnesium - 80, Potassium - 106, Sodium - 32, Iron - 57, Copper - 42, Manganese - 83, Zinc - 41, Selenium - 69, Chromium - 42.

✳ *Tomato Pâté*

Serves 16

Prepare the recipe for Vegetable Pâté with Velvet Sauce, doubling the ingredients. Steam the kale separately. Once all the basic ingredients have been mixed, divide the mixture in half. To one half add 3 fresh, peeled and seeded tomatoes, chopped (or 1 cup drained, chopped canned tomatoes), and 3 cloves garlic, minced.

Use two 8" x 8" baking pans. Using two thirds of the basic mixture, prepare one pâté in one pan. Use two thirds of the tomato mixture to prepare a second pâté, in the second pan. Add a layer of steamed fresh greens to each pâté then top these with the remaining tomato mixture. Bake, serve, and freeze as directed above.

Calories per serving (with 2 tablespoons Velvet Sauce): 515. Percent of calories from fat 12%, protein 24%, carbohydrate 63%, 1 mg cholesterol.

❉ *Three Bean Chili*

Serves 8

CHILI IS ONE OF OUR FAVORITES. WE USE EVEN MORE ONIONS AND UNLIM-ITED HOT SALSA. YOU COULD USE ADDITIONAL CHILI POWDER RATHER THAN GO THROUGH THE PROCESSING OF THE FRESH CHILES, BUT IT JUST WON'T HAVE THE SAME PUNCH AS THE REAL THING.

YOU MAY OMIT THE STEAK ENTIRELY AND SUFFER NO NUTRITIONAL SHORT-AGES HERE.

6 fresh jalapeño chiles
1 1/2 cups dried kidney beans,
    soaked overnight and drained
2/3 cup dried pinto beans,
    soaked overnight with kidney beans
2/3 cup dried soybeans,
    soaked overnight with kidney beans
6 cups chicken or vegetable broth
Olive oil cooking spray
3 medium-size onions, chopped
4 medium-size green bell peppers,
    seeded and chopped
8 fresh tomatoes, chopped
6 carrots, sliced into 1/4" rounds
3 strips (each 3" x 1") kombu,
    soaked for 15 minutes and chopped
3 to 4 cloves garlic, sliced in half
1 pound flank steak, trimmed of fat,
    cut into 1/2" pieces
2 cups chopped parsley
1/3 cup brewer's yeast
1/2 cup bran flakes
Half of a 6-ounce can tomato paste
1/2 cup water
1/4 cup ground cumin
1/3 cup chili powder
1/4 cup chopped fresh oregano or 2 teaspoons dried

**Hot or mild salsa (see the recipe for
Chicken Fajitas with Fresh Salsa**

Using rubber gloves, remove the stems and seeds from the chiles. Boil for 20 minutes in a small amount of water. Remove and discard the skins, then blend the flesh into a pulp in a blender. Set aside.

Cook the soaked and drained kidney beans, pinto beans and soybeans in the broth for one hour. Meanwhile, spray a large skillet with olive oil and sauté half of the onions, tomatoes, green bell peppers, and carrots for 10 minutes, stirring frequently. Transfer to a large bowl and sauté the remaining vegetables, then add all the vegetables to the beans along with the kombu.

Wipe out the skillet and spray with oil. Add a few cloves of garlic and the steak and sear over high heat. Add to the bean mixture along with the chile pulp, parsley, yeast, and bran.

Thin the tomato paste with the 1/2 cup of water and add to the beans. Add the cumin, chili powder, and oregano and simmer for at least 20 minutes. Serve with salsa.

To freeze: Ladle chili into freezerware dishes. Thaw overnight in the refrigerator and reheat in a saucepan or in the microwave.

Calories per serving: 575. Percent of calories from fat 30%, protein 49%, carbohydrates 25%, 31 mg cholesterol.

Nutritional profile (% of RDA) per serving: Vitamin A - 135, Vitamin C - 185, Vitamin D - 103, Vitamin E - 111, Vitamin K - 154, Thiamine - 252, Riboflavin - 74, Niacin - 73, Vitamin B6 - 113, Folacin - 210, Vitamin B12 - 132, Pantothenic Acid - 86, Biotin - 36, Calcium - 24, Phosphorus - 84, Magnesium - 81, Potassium - 155, Sodium - 34, Iron - 80, Copper - 61, Manganese - 76, Zinc - 58, Selenium - 75, Chromium - 101.

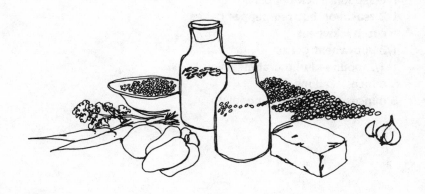

✳ *Cioppino*

Serves 8

We have visited many restaurants in Los Angeles to compare cioppino and bouillabaisse. We still prefer the recipe below. Most commercial sauces are thick and heavy. This lighter cioppino preserves the bright taste of tomatoes, while featuring chunky pieces of fresh fish.

1 pound mussels, in shells
8 ounces clams, in shells
1 1/2 pounds black sea bass fillets
3 large stalks celery
1 large onion
2 pounds fresh plum tomatoes, seeded
1 pound fresh shiitake mushrooms
1 pound kale
1 1/2 pounds brussels sprouts
Olive oil cooking spray
8 large cloves garlic, minced
2 quarts vegetable broth
4 strips (each 3" x 1") kombu,
   soaked for 15 minutes and chopped
1 can (16 ounces) no-oil tomato sauce
1/2 cup chopped fresh parsley
   plus additional for garnish
2 tablespoons chopped fresh basil
1 tablespoon fresh oregano
1 teaspoon dried thyme
1 teaspoon dried rosemary
2 bay leaves
1 teaspoon black pepper
1/2 teaspoon hot red pepper flakes
1 cup buckwheat
1/3 cup wheat germ
1 1/2 pounds lump crabmeat
8 ounces scallops
8 ounces whole-wheat noodles

Scrub the mussels but do not remove the beards until just before cooking. Shell the clams. Cut the sea bass into bite-size pieces. Coarsely chop all the vegetables except for the brussels sprouts; cut these in half.

Spray a large skillet with olive oil. Lightly brown the garlic over medium heat, stirring often to prevent scorching. Add 3 cups of the vegetable broth, the kombu, and all the vegetables except the tomatoes, and cook until tender. Add the tomatoes and cook 10 minutes more. Add the tomato sauce, all the herbs, the pepper and pepper flakes, and the remaining broth. Bring to a simmer.

Add the buckwheat, cover, and continue cooking 15 minutes, then add the wheat germ, sea bass, mussels, clams, crab, and scallops. Cover and cook 10 to 12 minutes, until all the seafood is done. Discard any mussels that do not open.

In a separate pot, cook the noodles according to package instructions. Drain and add to the cioppino last. Remove the bay leaves and garnish with additional parsley to serve.

To freeze: Freeze promptly in freezerware dishes. Thaw overnight in the refrigerator and reheat in a medium-size saucepan or in the microwave.

Calories per serving: 550. Percent of calories from fat 19%, protein 61%, carbohydrates 20%, 157 mg cholesterol.

Nutritional profile (% of RDA) per serving: Vitamin A - 164, Vitamin C - 302, Vitamin D - 136, Vitamin E - 94, Vitamin K - 613, Thiamine - 75, Riboflavin - 59, Niacin - 68, Vitamin B6 - 97, Folacin - 50, Vitamin B12 - 491, Pantothenic Acid - 73, Biotin - 10, Calcium - 33, Phosphorus - 77, Magnesium - 98, Potassium - 211, Sodium - 76, Iron - 63, Copper - 23, Manganese - 61, Zinc - 38, Selenium - 318, Chromium - 90.

✳ *Pizza*

Serves 4

Everybody's favorite! Conventional pizza, though nutritious, is an extremely high-fat food. This pizza is extremely low-fat, filling, and flavorful, and fulfills the better part of your Recommended Daily Allowances for the day. The rice crust is as tasty as conventional pizza crust, and it carries 30 percent of the nutritional value in this recipe. If you store precooked rice in your freezer, you can save time in many of our recipes.

If you are a bread maker and prefer a regular wheat and yeast crust, use a whole-wheat, no-oil bread recipe, and be sure to add at least 1/4 cup of wheat germ, some brewer's yeast, and bran flakes to meet megameal Recommended Daily Allowance requirements.

Including the crust, the main nutritional boosters in this dish are the mushrooms for vitamin D, and of course the broccoli and beans. Apart from these, any assortment of vegetables can be used, making this a simple and creative venture. Canned beans and leftover steamed vegetables are time savers as well.

For variety, look at the Santa Fe Pizza. It uses many of the same ingredients, with salsa instead of tomato sauce, and the addition of extra-lean ground beef.

<u>Topping</u>
    1 cup nonfat spaghetti sauce or tomato sauce
    1/2 cup white beans,
        soaked overnight and drained
    1/4 cup soy beans,
        soaked with the white beans
    1 small eggplant
    Salt
    8 ounces fresh mushrooms, washed
    1/4 cup balsamic vinegar
    1 teaspoon dijon mustard
    1 clove garlic, minced
    1/4 teaspoon black pepper
    1 stalk broccoli, flowerets only

1 carrot, sliced into 1/2" rounds
1 sheet (4" x 2") nori, cut up fine
1/3 cup grated low-fat or nonfat mozzarella
1/4 cup black olives
    (optional, will add 30 calories per slice)

<u>Crust</u>
2 egg whites
1 1/4 cups cooked brown rice
1/2 cup grated sweet potato
1 heaping tablespoon brewer's yeast
1/4 cup wheat germ
1/3 cup bran flakes
1 teaspoon black pepper
Dried herbs of your choice
    (such as oregano and marjoram), to taste
Canola oil cooking spray

Preheat the broiler.

Cover the soaked, drained beans with water in a saucepan and bring to a boil over a low heat. Simmer, covered, for 45 minutes. Add water as necessary.

Meanwhile, slice the eggplant into 1/2" rounds. Sprinkle both sides of each round with salt, heap in a bowl, and let stand 10 minutes to leach out any bitter liquids. While they stand, trim the mushrooms and marinate them in a mixture of the vinegar, mustard, garlic, and pepper for 15 minutes, stirring to coat each cap.

Thoroughly wash all the salt off the eggplant; drain the mushrooms. Place a roasting rack in a flat roasting pan, spray with Canola oil and arrange the eggplant slices and mushrooms on it. Add 1 inch of water to the pan. Broil the eggplant and mushrooms for about 4 minutes, removing the mushrooms as the eggplant browns. Turn the eggplant over to brown on both sides. The mushrooms will finish before the eggplant, so watch closely; remove them while they are still round and plump. Once the eggplant cools, slice into long, thin strips.

Switch the heat in the oven from broil to bake and set the baking temperature at 400°F.

Prepare the crust: In a large bowl, lightly beat the egg whites.

Add the cooked rice, sweet potato, yeast, wheat germ, and bran flakes. Add pepper and herbs to your taste, oregano and marjoram being our favorites. Mix thoroughly. Spray a nonstick cookie sheet or pizza pan with canola oil. Press the rice mixture firmly into a large, 14" or 16" round. (The back of a plastic spatula works well for this. If the crust sticks to the utensil, rinse the utensil off with warm water.) Bake the crust for 15 minutes.

Meanwhile, thoroughly drain and cool the beans. Steam the broccoli and carrots.

Remove the crust from the oven, leaving the heat on at 400°F. Spread the chopped nori and beans evenly over the crust and spoon the tomato sauce over all, leaving 1/4" of crust clear around the edges. Artistically place the eggplant strips, mushroom caps, broccoli, and carrots over the sauce. Top with cheese and the optional olives and bake in the oven for 15 minutes. Serve hot.

To freeze: Plastic wrap each slice tightly in freezer paper or plastic wrap. Several slices can be layered together in larger freezer baggies. Individual servings will thaw in several hours. To reheat, wrap each slice in aluminum foil and bake in an oven preheated to 350°F for 15 minutes.

Calories per serving (without olives): 309. Percent of calories from fat 15%, protein 23%, carbohydrates 62%, 5 mg cholesterol.

Nutritional profile (% of RDA) per serving: Vitamin A - 122, Vitamin C - 114, Vitamin D - 16, Vitamin E - 72, Vitamin K - 225, Thiamine - 95, Riboflavin - 39, Niacin - 32, Vitamin B6 - 66, Folacin - 75, Vitamin B12 - 30, Pantothenic Acid - 60, Biotin - 21, Calcium - 16, Phosphorus - 39, Magnesium - 36, Potassium - 61, Sodium - 14, Iron - 34, Copper - 29, Manganese - 62, Zinc - 24, Selenium - 56, Chromium - 52.

✳ Santa Fe Pizza

Serves 4

Please read the introduction to Pizza. This pizza is a little simpler in that it replaces the pizza's eggplant and mushrooms with ground beef, hence there is no broiling. If you prefer a meat-free Santa Fe pizza, substitute vegetables for the meat in the Pizza recipe and prepare them according to that recipe.

To save time, use healthfully prepared (which means no lard) canned refried beans and bottled salsa.

Be as creative with these as you want. Shredded chicken or turkey could replace the beef. Try kidney beans instead of black beans (the soybeans must stay, however, to meet Megameal Recommended Daily Allowance requirements). Add additional salsa, orange slices, or whatever inspires you.

> 1/2 cup dried black beans,
>   soaked overnight and drained
> 1/4 cup dried soy beans,
>   soaked with the black beans
> 2 strips (each 3" x 1") kombu,
>   soaked for 15 minutes and chopped
> 2 stalks broccoli, flowerets only
> 1 red bell pepper, seeded and cut into thin strips
> Canola oil cooking spray
> 2 cloves garlic, pressed
> 1/2 cup chopped onion
> 2 ounces extra lean ground beef
>   or turkey, preferably white meat
> Crust ingredients as for Pizza
> 1 jar (12 ounces) bottled salsa, or use fresh
> 1 teaspoon dried oregano
> 1 teaspoon ground cumin
> Dash of salt and pepper
> 1/3 cup grated low fat or nonfat muenster,
>   Monterey jack, or cheddar cheese
> Additional ingredients for topping as desired (optional)

Preheat the oven to 400°F.

Cover the soaked, drained beans with water in a saucepan. (The soybeans will turn black, but since the beans will be pureed together, this doesn't matter.) Add the kombu and bring to a boil over low heat. Simmer, covered, for 45 minutes. Add water as necessary.

Cut the broccoli flowerets into bite-size pieces and steam for 8 minutes, or until crisp yet tender. Add the red bell pepper to the broccoli halfway through steaming.

Spray a small skillet with olive oil and brown the garlic and chopped onion for a few minutes over low heat, stirring frequently. Add the beef or turkey, stirring to separate and cook the meat evenly. Cook briefly, until the juices run clear and there is no pink meat showing. Remove from the heat.

Prepare and bake the crust as instructed.

Meanwhile, drain the beans. Puree in a food processor along with 1/4 cup of the salsa and the oregano, cumin, salt, and pepper. Remove the crust from the oven, leaving the heat at 400°F.

Coat the crust evenly with a thick layer of the beans. Cover with the remaining salsa, allowing 1/4 inch of beans to peek out around the edge. Spread the meat mixture on top of the salsa, then alternate the red pepper strips with the broccoli over the meat. Cover the pizza with cheese and bake for 15 minutes.

Serve hot, as is, or covered with chopped lettuce, onions, tomatoes, more salsa, thin slices of avocado, and dollops of low-fat or non-fat yogurt. Except for the avocado, these added toppings are so low in calories as to be virtually calorie free.

To freeze: Follow the freezing and reheating directions for pizza in the previous recipe. However, the added toppings for this Santa Fe pizza should be added fresh.

Calories per serving: 343. Percent of calories from fat 19%, protein 25%, carbohydrates 55%, 17 mg cholesterol.

Nutritional profile (% of RDA) per serving: Vitamin A - 80, Vitamin C - 122, Vitamin D - 12, Vitamin E - 72, Vitamin K - 202, Thiamine - 95, Riboflavin - 34, Niacin - 29, Vitamin B6 - 65, Folacin - 77, Vitamin B12 - 39, Pantothenic Acid - 48, Biotin - 20, Calcium - 16, Phosphorus - 39, Magnesium - 34, Potassium - 53, Sodium - 14, Iron - 33, Copper

- 21, Manganese - 59, Zinc - 28, Selenium - 51, Chromium - 57.

✳ *The Meganutrient Shake*

Serves 1

THE MEGANUTRIENT SHAKE CAN BE MEASURED OUT THE NIGHT BEFORE AND BLENDED FRESH FOR BREAKFAST. FRUITS CAN VARY, ALTHOUGH WE DO SUGGEST USING HALF A BANANA FOR TEXTURE AND AN ORANGE FOR VITAMIN C. AND WHILE ORANGES, BANANAS, AND APPLES ARE AVAILABLE YEAR LONG, SUMMER FRUITS OFFER GREATER VARIETY. HALF A MANGO, FOR INSTANCE, WILL BOOST YOUR VITAMIN A QUOTA BY 40 PERCENT AND FULFILL 50 PERCENT OF YOUR NEED FOR VITAMIN C, AND HALF A CUP OF STRAWBERRIES ADDED TO YOUR SHAKE WILL ADD 20 PERCENT OF YOUR FIBER REQUIREMENTS. YOU MAY SUBSTITUTE NONFAT DRY MILK AND WATER IF YOU RUN OUT OF SKIM MILK, OR TRY FROZEN ORANGE JUICE CONCENTRATE (ALTHOUGH THE REAL FRUIT BRINGS YOU FIBER AS WELL AS VITAMINS).

YOU MAY CHOOSE TO SUBSTITUTE 2 GRAMS NORI (1 PIECE 4" x 4") FOR THE BREWER'S YEAST. WHILE THEY PROVIDE APPROXIMATELY THE SAME AMOUNT OF IRON, YEAST IS HIGHER IN NIACIN.

1 cup nonfat (skim) milk
1/2 cup plain nonfat yogurt
1 orange, peeled and seeded
1/2 banana
4 dried apricots,
    plumped in water overnight and drained
1 tablespoon wheat germ
1 scant teaspoon brewer's yeast

Place all the ingredients in a blender and whip for several minutes.

Note: When you add 1 tablespoon of bran flakes, you gain 20 percent of your daily need for vitamin B12, 10 percent for vitamin A, and 10 percent for iron. The bran flakes make the shake almost thick enough to eat with a spoon, depending on what other fruits you use! One half of a mango boosts the shake by 119 percent of your daily need for vitamin A, 71 percent for vitamin C, and with 10 percent of your daily needs for fiber.

Calories per serving: 388. Percent of calories from fat 8%, protein 21%, carbohydrates 70%, 12 mg cholesterol.

Nutritional profile (% of RDA) per serving: Vitamin A - 38, Vitamin C - 176, Vitamin D - 26, Vitamin E - 43, Vitamin K - 35, Thiamine - 124, Riboflavin - 66, Niacin - 25, Vitamin B6 - 50, Folacin - 107, Vitamin B12 - 55, Pantothenic Acid - 83, Biotin - 24, Calcium - 51, Phosphorus - 56, Magnesium - 33, Potassium - 90, Sodium - 23, Iron - 16, Copper - 36, Manganese - 32, Zinc - 28, Selenium - 54, Chromium - 53.

Chapter 11

Free-Choice Recipes

Breakfasts

✳ Baked Apple

Serves 2

PREPARE THIS THE NIGHT BEFORE AND BAKE IT WHILE YOU SHOWER. PACK IT AS A LUNCH OR SERVE IT AS A DESSERT. ANY WAY YOU GO, MORNING, NOON OR NIGHT, THIS BAKED APPLE FILLS THE BILL. HALVE EACH APPLE AND YOU HAVE A LOW-CALORIE SALAD OR SNACK. SERVE IT COOL WITH A DOLLOP OF YOGURT MIXED WITH A LITTLE HONEY AND CHOPPED FRESH MINT. OR SERVE AS A SIDE DISH WITH LAMB OR TURKEY.

WE ARE TAKING A SHORTCUT BY USING A PREPARED, FORTIFIED CEREAL.

2 large Granny Smith or
    Rome Beauty apples
2/3 cup Grape Nuts
1/4 cup wheat germ
1 tablespoon raisins, chopped
Canola oil cooking spray

Wash and core both apples, removing approximately 1/2 cup of flesh from each apple. Mix together the Grape Nuts, wheat germ, and raisins.

Cut two large squares of heavy-duty aluminum foil. Overlap and crimp the edges of each to form a small casserole dish. Spray the insides with canola oil. Set each apple in its "dish" and fill with the cereal mixture. Seal the apples by crimping the foil over the top.

Set wrapped apples in the oven and bake for 30 minutes at 350°F. Allow to cool briefly or completely before serving.

Or you may microwave these apples. Set each apple in a small bowl or microwave-safe dish, and cover with vented microwavable plastic wrap. Use the bake or medium setting for 7 minutes, then leave apples in the microwave for an additional minute.

Serve either hot or cooled.

Calories per serving: 330. Percentage of calories from fat 4%, protein 10%, carbohydrates 86%, 0 mg cholesterol.

✳ *French Toast*

Serves 4

BAKING INSTEAD OF FRYING **F**RENCH TOAST WILL REDUCE YOUR FAT INTAKE. **W**HAT YOU MAY NOT EXPECT, HOWEVER, IS WHAT LIGHT AND FLUFFY SLICES YOU'LL BE SERVING!

Canola oil cooking spray
8 slices light (not dense,
    heavy, whole-grain) whole-wheat bread
1 cup evaporated skim milk
1 whole egg plus 4 egg whites,
    or eight ounces soft tofu
1/4 cup wheat germ
1 teaspoon honey
1 teaspoon vanilla
Dash each of cinnamon and salt
Any fresh fruit, chopped to use as a topping

Preheat oven to 350°F.

Spray a 13"x 9" baking pan with canola oil. Arrange the bread slices in the pan, making 2 layers if necessary. Combine all the remaining ingredients except the fruit and beat well, or whip in a food processor, especially if using tofu.

Pour the mixture over the bread, cover, and let "marinate" for 20 minutes or in the refrigerator overnight.

Bake for 30 to 40 minutes, or until lightly browned. Serve with chopped fresh fruit or sprinkle with powdered sugar.

Calories per serving (without fruit): 216. Percentage of calories from fat 14%, protein 23%, carbohydrates 62%, 0 mg cholesterol.

✳ Buckwheat Pancakes

Makes 8 3-inch round pancakes; serves 4

PUREED FRUIT MIXED WITH A LITTLE NONFAT YOGURT AND HONEY MAKES A WONDERFUL TOPPING WITH THESE PANCAKES.

<u>Pancakes</u>
1/3 cup buckwheat flour
1/4 cup whole-wheat flour
3 tablespoons wheat germ
2 teaspoons baking powder
Dash of salt
1 egg, beaten
1 teaspoon honey
1/2 cup buttermilk
1/4 cup apple juice
Canola oil cooking spray

<u>Topping</u>
1 cup fresh fruit,
    coarsely chopped or whole berries
3/4 cup plain nonfat yogurt
1 teaspoon honey

Combine the dry ingredients thoroughly and set aside. Combine the liquids and whip vigorously with a fork until thoroughly blended. Add the liquids to the flours and stir to moisten. You should have a lumpy batter. Do not overmix; the lumps will disappear as the pancakes cook.

Spray a griddle or a large skillet with canola oil, then heat over medium heat until hot.

Spoon 2 large tablespoons of batter into the center of the griddle and, in a swirling motion, lift the griddle to distribute the batter into a slightly larger pancake. Turn the pancakes when bubbles form. Repeat to use up the remaining batter.

To make the topping, puree the fruit with the honey in a food processor. Add the yogurt and blend for 30 seconds. Serve with the pancakes.

Calories per serving (with topping): 170. Percentage of calories from fat 12%, protein 12%, carbohydrates 73%; 68 mg cholesterol.

✳ *Scrambled Eggs with Variations*

Serves 4

IF YOU HAVE BEEN WATCHING YOUR CHOLESTEROL, YOU PROBABLY KNOW ABOUT SCRAMBLED EGG WHITES. YOU MAY NOT YET HAVE TRIED SCRAMBLED TOFU! THE FOLLOWING RECIPES ARE A BASIC FOUNDATION FOR ANY NUMBER OF VEGETABLE COMBINATIONS. SEE CHAPTER 9 FOR USES FOR LEFTOVER RAW OR COOKED EGGS YOLKS.

Scrambled Eggs	Scrambled Egg Whites with Mushrooms
Olive oil cooking spray	Olive oil cooking spray
2 whole eggs plus 4 egg whites	5 egg whites
1/4 small onion, minced	4 fresh mushrooms, chopped
1/2 tomato, chopped	1/4 small onion, minced
2 tablespoons	1/2 fresh tomato, chopped
minced fresh parsley	1/2 teaspoon dried tarrago
Dash of black pepper	1/2 teaspoon
	minced fresh basil

Scrambled Tofu with Garlic
and Red Peppers
Olive oil cooking spray
6 ounces soft tofu
2 fresh mushrooms, chopped
1/4 small onion, minced
1/4 red bell pepper, seeded and chopped
1/2 clove garlic, pressed
1/2 teaspoon each ground turmeric
   and dried thyme
Dash of black pepper

For all variations, spray a medium-size skillet with olive oil and place over low heat. Add the vegetables of choice, cover, and allow to "poach" in their own juices for 2 to 3 minutes. Add the herbs and spices. Dry-fry, stirring a few times, until the vegetables are soft.

If using the egg whites and/or egg, beat lightly. With a wooden or plastic spoon, stir the eggs into the vegetable mixture and scramble light to firm, as you prefer. If using tofu, add to the vegetables along with the herbs and spices. Break the wedge of tofu up into chunky pieces while "scrambling." Tabasco sauce is quite good with tofu!

Calories per serving scrambled whole eggs (with added whites): 117. Percentage of calories from fat 45%, protein 39%, carbohydrates 15%, 137 mg cholesterol.

Calories per serving scrambled whites with mushrooms: 45. Percentage of calories from fat 4%, protein 55%, carbohydrates 42%, 0 mg cholesterol.

Calories per serving scrambled tofu with garlic and red peppers: 102. Percentage of calories from fat 40%, protein 37%, carbohydrates 23%, 0 mg cholesterol.

✳ Cream of Wheat, Oat, or Corn

Serves 1

THERE ARE MANY "CREAM OF" CEREALS ON THE MARKET TODAY. AND AT FIRST GLANCE, THEY APPEAR TO BE NUTRITIOUS. HOWEVER HERALDED AS BEING HIGH IN FIBER, MOST OF THESE ARE NOT. ONE CUP (100 G) OF HOT WHOLE WHEAT CEREAL CONTAINS ONLY 2 GRAMS OF FIBER, WHILE 1 SMALL PEAR CONTAINS 1.5 GRAMS, AND 2 TABLESPOONS OF RAISINS 1.3 GRAMS OF FIBER. ONE DAY TAKE A FEW EXTRA MOMENTS TO READ THE LABELS ON THE CEREAL BOXES IN YOUR LOCAL MARKET. MOST OF THE "HIGH IN FIBER" LABELS CONTAIN LITTLE MORE THAN A CUP OF WHOLE WHEAT. 100% ALL FIBER CEREAL AND BRAN FLAKES ARE TWO EXCEPTIONS, CONTAINING 12 GRAMS EACH IN A CUP OF CEREAL. IT PAYS TO READ YOUR LABELS!

OAT, WHEAT, AND NOW CORN BRAN ARE ALL EXTREMELY HIGH IN FIBER. A FEW YEARS AGO THE SOLUBLE FORM OF FIBER FOUND IN THE GREATEST DENSITY IN OAT BRAN WAS CONSIDERED TO BE THE HEALTHIEST FOR LOWERING BLOOD CHOLESTEROL. HOWEVER, NOW IT IS BELIEVED THAT ALL FORMS OF GRAIN BRANS WILL HELP IN LOWERING BLOOD CHOLESTEROL. EITHER OAT, WHEAT, OR CORN BRAN, OR A COMBINATION, WOULD WORK WELL IN THIS RECIPE.

    1/3 cup oat bran
    1/2 cup apple or peach juice
    1/2 cup low-fat milk
    1 tablespoon wheat germ
    1 teaspoon maple syrup
    2 teaspoons raisins
    2 walnut halves, chopped

Combine the bran, juice, milk, wheat germ, and maple syrup in a small saucepan. Heat over a low flame until the mixture boils, stirring constantly to prevent lumping. Cook over low heat for 3 minutes.

Remove from the heat and cover. Let stand 1 minute. Gently stir in the raisins and walnuts.

Calories per serving: 200. Percentage of calories from fat 17%, protein 10%, carbohydrates 72%, 1 mg cholesterol.

Soups

✳ Orange Vegetable Soup

Serves 4

THIS SOUP IS LOADED WITH FLAVOR AND NUTRIENTS BOTH. ITS COLOR IS HARVEST ORANGE, A BRIGHT SIGN OF ITS SUPER VITAMIN A BOOST. A STRONG ANTIOXIDANT, VITAMIN A IS IN THE FRONT BATTALION AGAINST FREE RADICALS. SERVE WITH THE BEANS-AND-GREENS SALAD FOR A LIGHT MEAL. OR SERVE ALONG WITH SALMON OR A SLICE OF VEGETABLE QUICHE (PAGE 142).

1 large sweet potato, peeled
2 carrots
1 cup water
1/4 cup barley
2 cups cooked pumpkin (fresh or canned)
2 strips (each 3" x 1") kombu,
 soaked in 1/2 cup water for 10 minutes
 and coarsely chopped
2 cups vegetable broth
1 tablespoon brewer's yeast
2 tablespoons whole-wheat flour
2 tablespoons wheat germ
1 tablespoon dried rosemary
1 teaspoon marjoram
2 tablespoons ground cumin
1 tablespoon ground ginger
1/2 teaspoon black pepper, or to taste

Salt to taste
1 orange, peeled and seeded

Cut the sweet potato and carrot into 2" chunks, then steam until soft, approximately 10 minutes.

In a medium saucepan heat the 1 cup water to a boil. Add the barley and simmer covered over low heat for 15 minutes.

In a food processor, combine half each of the sweet potato, carrots and pumpkin with the kombu and a little of the broth. Puree until smooth. Add the other half of the vegetables, the barley, yeast, whole-wheat flour, wheat germ, herbs and spices, orange, and half the remaining broth. The soup will be very thick. While the motor is running, gently pour in the remaining broth until the soup reaches the consistency you prefer. If you like a creamier texture, you may want to further purée the soup in several small batches in a blender. Season with salt to taste, reheat, and serve.

Calories per serving: 151. Percentage of calories from fat 4.5%, protein 12%, carbohydrates 83%, 0 mg cholesterol.

✳ *Split Pea Soup*

Serves 8

In India, split pea and lentil soups are an integral part of almost every meal. The variety of lentils, spices, and vegetables added to these soups is limited only by your imagination. This version is hearty and satisfying yet light. On a cold night, this soup goes well with some cornbread or roasted chicken.

5 cups chicken or vegetable broth (or water)
1 cup dried split peas
1/4 cup finely chopped kombu,
    soaked for 30 minutes to soften
1 teaspoon ground turmeric
1/2 teaspoon ground coriander

1 teaspoon peeled and grated fresh ginger
Salt to taste
1 pound fresh spinach, washed and coarsely chopped,
    or 1 package (10 ounces) frozen, thawed
1/4 teaspoon olive oil
1 clove garlic
2 teaspoons cumin seeds
1 teaspoon paprika

In a heavy 3-quart saucepan bring the broth, split peas, kombu, turmeric, coriander, and ginger to a full boil over high heat, stirring occasionally. Reduce the heat to low, cover, and simmer for 1 hour or until the peas are soft.

Remove from the heat and add salt to taste. Add the spinach, cover, and return to the heat. Boil gently for 8 to 10 minutes. Frozen spinach will need only reheating, not cooking.

In a small skillet heat the oil. When it is hot, add the garlic and cumin seeds and fry until they are brown, stirring constantly. Add the paprika, stir, and then pour the spice mixture into the soup. Cover the soup and let the spices soak into it for a few minutes before serving.

Calories per serving: 124. Percentage of calories from fat 17%, protein 24%, carbohydrates 59%, 0 mg cholesterol.

❋ Split Pea Soup with Bananas

Serves 8

THE RICHNESS OF BANANA IN THIS VARIATION MAKES IT ESPE-
CIALLY FILLING!

Prepare the soup as in Split Pea Soup, above, but halfway through cooking the peas, add 1 cup thinly sliced radishes and 2 green (under-ripe) bananas, peeled and sliced into 1/4" rounds. If desired, add 1 to 2 green chilies, seeded and minced, to the split peas along with the spinach. Add 1 tablespoon lemon juice just before serving.

✳ *Creole Gumbo*

Serves 8

WE HAVE PROVIDED YOU, IN THIS MEAL, WITH HEALTH CHOICES. IF YOU ARE A VEGETARIAN, OR REDUCING YOUR MEAT CONSUMPTION, THEN REST ASSURED THAT TOFU BOOSTS THE CALCIUM CONTENT OF THIS MEAL BY 50 PERCENT, WHICH NEITHER CHICKEN NOR FISH WILL, WHILE IT ELIMINATES CHOLESTEROL. WHEN COMPARING PROTEIN CONTENT BETWEEN TOFU, CHICKEN, AND SHRIMP, CHICKEN WINS HANDS DOWN WITH 265% OF YOUR RECOMMENDED DAILY ALLOWANCE, SHRIMP WITH 172%, AND TOFU WITH 122%. BUT ANY OF THE THREE IS MORE THAN ADEQUATE. SHRIMP IS HIGH IN CHOLESTEROL, ALTHOUGH IT IS HIGH-HDL, AND ALSO TRIPLES VITAMIN E, DOUBLES VITAMIN D (THE SEAWEED IN THIS SOUP SUPPLIES MORE THAN YOUR DAILY NEEDS FOR D), AND SUPPLIES ALL THE B12 YOU NEED FOR THE DAY. SHRIMP IS ALSO VERY HIGH IN SELENIUM. VEGETARIANS NEED PRIMARILY TO CONCERN THEMSELVES WITH B12. A GLASS OF SKIM MILK, YOGURT, OR HARD BOILED EGGS WILL FILL THE GAP.

THE WORD "GUMBO" IS SYNONYMOUS WITH OKRA. GUM ORIGINALLY MEANT A STICKY PLANT SECRETION (SIMILAR TO OKRA). THIS TEXTURE DISAPPEARS WITH COOKING.

2 small eggplants
Salt
1 1/2 cups water
1/3 cup brown rice
1/3 cup wild rice
1 pound okra, preferably fresh
1 teaspoon olive oil
10 cloves garlic, minced
2 large onions, chopped
2 large red or green bell peppers,
      seeded and diced
6 cups chicken or vegetable broth
2 teaspoons dried thyme
2 teaspoons paprika
1/4 teaspoon hot chili powder
1 sheet nori (4"x 2")

2/3 cup arame seaweed (roughly 2 ounces)
2 strips kombu (each 3" x 1"), chopped
2 packages (each 10 ounces) frozen corn
1 medium-size head cauliflower,
   broken into flowerets
4 medium-size fresh tomatoes, chopped
3 large, skinless, boneless chicken breasts,
   sliced into bite-size pieces
   or 1 pound medium-size shrimp, peeled
   or 1 pound extra firm tofu, sliced into bite-size pieces
Black pepper to taste
1 teaspoon cider vinegar (optional)
8 corn tortillas

Trim the stalk end of the eggplant. Cut into 1/2" cubes and place in a colander. Sprinkle about 1 teaspoon salt over the eggplant, and shake to distribute evenly. Let the eggplant "sweat" for 10 minutes, while you prepare the rice.

Heat the 1 1/2 cups water in a 2-quart saucepan. When the water boils, combine the wild and brown rices. Slowly pour into the boiling water. Reduce the heat to low, cover, and simmer for 45 minutes, or until all liquid has been absorbed.

Meanwhile, trim the stalk ends from the okra. Cut the okra into 1/2" pieces and set aside. Thoroughly rinse the eggplant under cold water and drain well.

In a large kettle heat the olive oil. Add the garlic, onion, bell pepper, and eggplant. Stir quickly until all the vegetables have been coated with a little oil. Add a little of the broth and sauté over low heat for 5 minutes. Stir in the spices and cook gently for a few minutes.

Add the remaining broth, nori, arame, kombu, corn, cauliflower, tomatoes, and chicken, or tofu. Cover and simmer gently for 20 minutes. The last 10 minutes of cooking, add the okra. The okra should be bright green and just barely cooked. It becomes slippery and dull when overcooked.

Add the rice and simmer for a few minutes. If you are using shrimp, add, along with the vinegar, with the rice and simmer for 5 minutes, stirring occasionally.

Meanwhile, heat the corn tortillas, by wrapping in aluminum foil to keep them soft and place them in a toaster oven. Season the gumbo with salt and pepper, and serve with the hot tortillas.

Calories per serving: 396. Percentage of calories from fat 10%, protein 31%, carbohydrates 59%, 55 mg cholesterol.

✳ *Chicken Noodle Soup*

Serves 8

OFTEN THE SIMPLEST AND MOST TRADITIONAL FOODS SATISFY THE PALATE, THE BODY, AND THE SOUL. CHICKEN NOODLE SOUP CONJURES UP MEMORIES OF LAPTOP BLANKETS AND WARM FIRES — THINGS THAT MAKE US FEEL GOOD. THIS SOUP CAN HAVE A MOST UNUSUAL KICK TO IT IF YOU CHOOSE TO ADD THE CHILI, AND IT'S VERY SIMPLE TO PREPARE.

SERVE THE SOUP WITH A HEARTY GREEN SALAD AND/OR A SLICE OF WHOLE-GRAIN TOAST.

8 cups water
1 pound skinless, boneless chicken breasts,
    cut into bite-size pieces
1/2 bunch celery,
    preferably the heart with the leaves, diced
1 bunch carrots, sliced into 1/2-inch rounds
    1 bunch broccoli, flowerets only
5 ounces string beans,
    trimmed and sliced into bite-size pieces
6 to 7 kale leaves or
    1 bunch spinach, washed and chopped
1 Anaheim chile (optional), seeded and minced
4 ounces rice elbow noodles,
    or whole-wheat elbows
1 tablespoon dried marjoram
1 teaspoon coriander seed
Dash of salt

In a large dutch oven or kettle, bring the water to a boil. Add the chicken, all the vegetables, and the chile if using. Simmer over medium heat for 45 minutes.

Add the noodles, marjoram, coriander seed and salt and continue simmering another 12 minutes for rice noodles, 15 minutes or longer for whole wheat. Taste check the whole-wheat noodles to make sure that they are cooked. Add salt and seasonings to suit your palate.

Calories per serving: 200. Percentage of calories from fat 10%, protein 40%, carbohydrates 50%, 36 mg cholesterol.

✳ Miracle Soup

Serves 12, makes 4 1/2 quarts

THIS IS THE SOUP WE REFERRED TO AS THE "IN-BETWEEN MEALS" SOUP. IT'S RICH IN FLAVOR AND THE BROTH ALONE IS EXCELLENT IN GRAIN STUFFINGS.

3 leeks, well washed
1 large green bell pepper, seeded
1 small cauliflower
2 stalks broccoli
5 carrots
1/2 cup chopped parsley
12 cups water

Slice all the vegetables into 1-inch chunks. In a large pot, bring the water to a boil and add the vegetables. Simmer over low heat for 45 minutes.

This soup remains fresh for 5 days in the refrigerator.

Calories per serving: 35. Percentage of calories from fat 5%, protein 20%, carbohydrates 74%, 0 mg cholesterol.

❋ *Watercress Soup*

Serves 8

THIS COLD, GREEN, VITAMIN C-RICH SOUP USHERS IN THOSE REFRESHING SUMMER EVENINGS.

PUREED SOUPS MADE IN A FOOD PROCESSOR ARE OFTEN NOT QUITE SMOOTH ENOUGH TO PASS AS "CREAMY." IF YOU WANT A TRULY RICH, BUTTERY TEXTURE FOR THIS SOUP, ONCE THE WATERCRESS IS PUREED IN THE FOOD PROCESSOR, TRANSFER IT TO A BLENDER. A FEW SECONDS IN THE BLENDER AND THIS SOUP IS A CREAMED DELICACY.

3 bunches fresh watercress
1/2 medium-size red onion
1/4 cup cornstarch or arrowroot
1 teaspoon ground coriander
Dash of salt
11/2 cups chicken or vegetable broth
2 cups buttermilk or evaporated skim milk
1 teaspoon grated orange rind (optional)

Remove and discard the larger watercress stems. Place the leaves, onion, cornstarch, coriander, salt and 1 cup of the broth in a food processor or blender. Puree fully.

Pour the puree into a medium-size saucepan and add the rest of the broth. Heat over medium heat until the soup just boils. Reduce the heat to low and simmer for 8 to 10 minutes, stirring frequently. When the soup begins to thicken, slowly blend in the buttermilk. Remove from the heat and stir in the orange rind.

Cool for 1 hour before serving.

Calories per serving: 31. Percentage of calories from fat 17%, protein 30%, carbohydrates 53%, 2 mg cholesterol.

Grains

About Grains

We have largely been a meat and potato eating society, even though our country's ancestors savored indigenous grains such as corn, amaranth, and wheat. Grains have been delegated a secondary role on our menu.

In 1991 the U.S. Department of Agriculture (USDA) issued dietary guidelines to replace the 1977 recommendations of a Senate Select Committee on nutrition. Whereas the 1977 version said to "eat foods with adequate starch and fiber," the current guidelines say to "choose a diet with plenty of vegetables, fruits and grain products." Using a pyramid design to illustrate what the bulk of our diet should be, bread, cereal, rice and pasta foods form the base of the pyramid. Fats, oils and sweets are to be used very sparingly, and thus are at the narrowest portion of the pyramid, on top. We recommend that grains become the main event of most of your meals. Many of the One-A-Day Megameals are largely grains.

The following grains and recipes are but the beginning. Be inspired and experiment.

Amaranth: This contains the best balance of proteins of any grain. Used largely as a cereal, amaranth is sold as a very tiny, delicate seed. Amaranth flour is also wonderful to add to baked goods. Look for it in your health food store.

Barley: Similar in texture to an al dente pasta when cooked, with a mild nutty flavor. Barley comes from the grass family and undergoes a pearling process similar to rice, (the inedible husk of the grain is removed and discarded). Pearled barley boosts the amount of fiber.

When added to soups, barley can be used as a thickener by lengthening the cooking time. With fresh fruit, it makes a great breakfast dish.

Buckwheat groats (kasha): Buckwheat is actually a fruit in the rhubarb family! Yet you may treat it as a grain. It is featured herein with Buckwheat Pancakes.

Bulgur wheat: This is a form of wheat berry that has been precooked, dried, and cracked. Since it has been precooked, it cooks up quickly, and is high in insoluble fiber.

Cornmeal: Used in tamales and cornbread, corn (maize) is technically a grain. Cornmeal when cooked is not as high in fiber as bulgur wheat, but its many uses and rich, sweet flavor make it a favorite.

Couscous: Another precooked cracked-wheat product. Whole-wheat couscous is now available in many natural food stores. You will find couscous in the international section of the supermarket. Easy to digest, couscous makes a wonderful light meal any time of the day. It cooks up in less than 10 minutes and can be used in place of other grains for pilafs, stir-fries, and stuffings.

Millet: Nutritionally one of the best grains, millet has one of the most complete proteins of all grains, being low in lysine only. Complement it with a small portion of dairy, beans, meats, fish, poultry, wheat germ or bran for a highly nutritious meal.

Millet is a round, yellow, seed-like grain that cooks like rice but in half the time. With 287 calories in a cup of cooked millet compared to 216 in a cup of rice, 10 grams of protein and only 3 grams of fat, millet tops the grain list as a superfood. It has a nutty, subtle flavor and is equally good for breakfast, dessert or as a side dish in place of rice.

Oats: We are familiar with oatmeal for breakfast, and in cookies. And oat bran has headlined every nutritional column. While oat bran is higher in soluble fiber than wheat bran, the jury is still out as to whether soluble fiber is indeed the agent that it is now thought to lower blood cholesterol.

Rice, brown: Brown rice simply is nutritionally superior to white rice. In many countries rice is the mainstay of the diet. The Japanese consider a meal incomplete without rice, which they eat even for breakfast. When mixed with beans, spinach, cauliflower, or broccoli, rice forms a complete protein.

Rice, wild: Wild rice is technically not a grain but a tall aquatic grass. Adding it to rice dishes will lighten them up, the "grain" being larger and less dense then rice.

Wheat berries: These whole-grain berries include the germ, bran, and endosperm of the wheat grain.

Cooking Times for Grains

Grain	Simmering Time	Quantity
Amaranth	About 25 minutes	1 part grain to 3 parts liquid
Barley	About 35 minutes	1 part grain to 2 parts liquid
Buckwheat	About 20 minutes	1 part grain to 2 parts liquid
Bulgur	About 15 minutes.	1 part grain to 2 parts liquid
Cornmeal	About 20 minutes	1 part grain to 3 parts liquid
Couscous	About 7 minutes	1 part grain to 1 1/2 parts liquid
Millet	About 20 minutes	1 part grain to 2 parts liquid
Oats	About 30 minutes	1 part cereal to 3 parts liquid
Rice, brown	About 40 minutes	1 part grain to 2 1/4 parts liquid
Rice, wild	About 40 minutes	1 part grain to 3 parts liquid
Wheat berries	About 1 hour*	1 part grain to 2 1/2 parts liquid

*and soak overnight in water to cover prior to cooking

✳ Couscous with Peas and Mint

Serves 4

2 1/2 cups vegetable or chicken broth
1 1/2 cups couscous, preferably whole-wheat
1 1/2 cups fresh or frozen peas
2 scallions, whites only, chopped fine
3 tablespoons finely chopped fresh mint

In a medium-size saucepan, bring the broth to a boil. Add the couscous, reduce the heat to low, cover, and simmer for 15 minutes.

Meanwhile, if using frozen peas, cook according to package directions. Fresh peas can be steamed for 8 minutes.

Fluff the couscous, add the scallions and mint, and mix together. Serve immediately.

Calories per serving: 180. Percentage of calories from fat 5%, protein 12%, carbohydrates 83%, 0 mg cholesterol.

✳ Spinach Rice Casserole

Serves 8

THIS IS SUCH A SURPRISINGLY SIMPLE AND GOOD DISH THAT YOU MAY JUST AS WELL DOUBLE THE RECIPE AND FREEZE SOME FOR THE FUTURE. ADD BROILED FISH, CHICKEN, OR A BOWL OF SPLIT PEA SOUP, ALONG WITH A BOWL OF NONFAT YOGURT AND FRUIT FOR DESSERT AND YOU WILL HAVE AMPLY NOURISHED YOURSELF!

3 cups water
2/3 cup wild rice
2/3 cup brown rice
Olive or canola oil cooking spray
2 cloves garlic, minced
1 medium-size onion, chopped
2 pounds fresh spinach, washed, drained, and chopped

2 eggs
1 cup low-fat or nonfat cottage cheese
1/2 cup nonfat (skim) milk
1 tablespoon brewer's yeast
1/4 cup fresh parsley, chopped
2 sheets (each 4"x 2") nori, chopped
Dried tarragon, thyme, and cayenne pepper to taste

Boil the 3 cups of water in a medium-size saucepan. Add the two rices, cover, reduce heat and simmer for 40 minutes.

Meanwhile, preheat the oven to 350°F. Spray an 8" x 8" baking pan with oil.

Spray a medium skillet with oil. Add the garlic and onion and stir-fry for 2 minutes. Add the spinach and cook another 2 minutes. Set aside.

In a large bowl mix together the eggs, cottage cheese, milk, yeast, parsley, nori, herbs, and cayenne. Add the rice and vegetables and mix all ingredients together thoroughly.

Press the rice mixture evenly into the prepared pan. Bake for 30 to 40 minutes, until the casserole no longer bubbles and all the juices have been absorbed.

Calories per serving: 300. Percentage of calories from fat 8%, protein 19%, carbohydrates 71%, 70 mg cholesterol.

✳ *Spiced Green Rice*

Serves 8

FOR YEARS I'VE PREPARED RICE AS A SIMPLE, NUTRITIOUS COMPLEX CAR-BOHYDRATE. ONLY RECENTLY, WHEN I BEGAN EXPLORING ETHNIC CUISINE, DID I DISCOVER THE INFINITE POSSIBILITIES TO DRESS UP A SIMPLE RICE DISH. THIS VERSION CAN BE SEASONED WITH HERBS ALONE FOR A MILDER ACCOMPANIMENT TO CURRIES, OR SPICED UP FOR STEAMED VEGETABLES, POULTRY, OR FISH. ADD DIFFERENT CHOPPED VEGETABLES AND HERBS TO CUSTOM-DESIGN THE RICE FOR YOUR OWN MEAL.

2 large cloves garlic, peeled
1 bunch fresh cilantro, leaves only
1/2 cup parsley leaves
1/4 cup chopped onion
1 sheet nori (optional), torn up
4 1/4 cups broth, chicken or vegetable
2 cups short grain brown rice
2 green bell peppers, roasted and chopped

Place the garlic, cilantro, parsley, onion, and nori in a food processor along with 1/4 cup of the broth. Process until finely chopped.

In a 2-quart pot, bring the remaining broth to a boil with the chopped herb blend. Slowly add the rice. Reduce the heat, cover, and simmer for 35 to 45 minutes, or until all the liquid has been absorbed. Gently stir in the green peppers to serve.

Calories per serving: 190. Percentage of calories from fat 5%, protein 10%, carbohydrates 85%, 0 mg cholesterol.

❋ Rice with Raisins, Peas, and Nuts

Serves 12

MIXED RICE AND BEAN DISHES ARE POPULAR IN THE SO-CALLED UNDER-DEVELOPED COUNTRIES. THIS IS DUE LARGELY TO THE EXPENSE AND UNAVAILABILITY OF MEAT AND FISH PROTEINS. YET THE DEVELOPED COUNTRIES ARE REALLY THE PAUPERS! FOR WE HAVE NOT CREATIVELY EXPLORED THE WIDE VARIETY OF NUTRITIONALLY RICH AND TASTEBUD-SATISFYING RICE AND BEAN DISHES. RICE AND BEANS FORM A COMPLETE PROTEIN, AND HENCE ARE A PERFECT ALTERNATIVE TO MEATS.

THE FOLLOWING RECIPE, AN ADAPTATION FROM A TRADITIONAL INDIAN DISH CALLED KHICHARI, IS A BASIC STARTER. YOU COULD CHANGE OR ADD ANY COMBINATION OF VEGETABLES, SEEDS, OR BEANS THAT YOU HAPPEN TO HAVE ON HAND. SPLIT PEAS, PREFERABLY THE YELLOW KIND, ARE AN IDEAL MIX IN THAT THEY COOK UP QUICKLY AND CAN THUS BE ADDED TO THE RICE DURING THE COOKING PROCESS. TRY THIS RECIPE BEFORE YOU SUBSTITUTE A LARGER BEAN,

WHICH WOULD HAVE TO BE COOKED PRIOR TO THE RICE.

PREPARING THE INGREDIENTS TAKES ONLY 15 MINUTES. THE SIMMERING TIME IS 45 MINUTES, WITH MINIMAL SUPERVISION.

11/2 cups brown rice
2 teaspoons ground turmeric
    mixed with 2 tablespoons water
Olive oil cooking spray
2 tablespoons cumin seeds
2 to 3 tablespoons dried hot pepper flakes
12 whole cloves
9 cups water
1 teaspoon onion powder
1 teaspoon garlic powder
1/3 cup chopped almonds,
    toasted and chopped
1/3 cup sunflower seeds, toasted with the almonds
1/3 cup golden raisins
Dash each of salt and black pepper
1/2 cup wheat germ
1 cup yellow split peas
1 1/2 cups frozen green peas

Preheat the oven to 300°F.

In a small bowl, combine the rice with half of the turmeric mixture. Mix thoroughly and set aside.

Spray a large heatproof casserole or kettle with olive oil. Over a medium heat add the cumin seeds, hot pepper flakes, and cloves. Stir for 1 minute, or until the seeds begin to toast. Do not allow to burn. Add the 9 cups water along with the onion and garlic powders. Bring to a rolling boil. Add the rice, almonds, sunflower seeds, raisins, salt, pepper, and wheat germ. Return to a gentle boil, then lower the heat, cover, and simmer for 20 minutes.

Stir the remaining turmeric mixture into the split peas and add to the half-cooked rice. Simmer for another 15 minutes, adding more water if necessary. Add the frozen peas and simmer for a final 10 minutes, adjusting the seasonings as necessary.

Serve hot.

Calories per serving: 300. Percentage of calories from fat 20%, protein 15%, carbohydrates 46%, 0 mg cholesterol.

✳ *Tabouleh*

Serves 8

Bulgur wheat is a versatile grain used much like rice in soups, pilafs, stuffings, and grain salads. Tabouleh comes to us from the Middle East and is frequently served with such delicious dishes as baba ganoush, hummus, and felafel.

This is a very easy recipe. The grain does not need to cook at all. It is soaked in water and then mixed with tomatoes and lots of parsley for a refreshingly light dish.

1 cup fine-grained bulgur wheat
3 cups water
2 large fresh tomatoes
1/2 onion, minced
2 cups fresh parsley, finely chopped
1/4 cup lemon juice
1 tablespoon olive oil
1/2 teaspoon black pepper
Dash of salt
Lettuce leaves or pita pockets

Soak the bulgur wheat in a large bowl with the 3 cups of water for 1 hour.

To seed and core the tomatoes, cut each one in half crosswise. With a grapefruit spoon (a small knife with a serrated edge will work, but the spoon is curved and has a serrated edge) gently dish out the seeds and internal membrane. Soak up any extra juice with paper towels. Chop the tomatoes into 1/4" pieces and set aside.

Drain the bulgur in a fine-mesh colander, pressing firmly with a large spoon to remove as much liquid as possible. Combine in a large bowl the bulgur, tomatoes, onion, parsley, lemon juice, olive oil, pep-

per, and salt. Mix thoroughly but gently, so as not to smash the tomatoes.

Serve over lettuce leaves or with pita pockets.

Calories per serving: 200. Percentage of calories from fat 11%, protein 11%, carbohydrates 78%, 0 mg cholesterol.

✳ Curried Two-Grain Salad

Serves 8, makes about 5 1/3 cups

DURING THE SPRING IN SOUTHERN CALIFORNIA, WE POTLUCK AND PICNIC
EXTENSIVELY. ALL OF THE GRAIN SALADS ARE EXCELLENT NOVELTIES ALONGSIDE
THE GENERAL OUTDOOR FARE, AND THEY COMPLEMENT BARBECUES ESPECIALLY
WELL. VIRTUALLY ANY STEAMED VEGETABLE COULD BE ADDED TO THESE MAR-
INATED DISHES.

WHEAT BERRIES ARE A HEARTY ALTERNATIVE TO RICE, AND YOU SHOULD BE
ABLE TO FIND THEM AT A HEALTH FOOD STORE. ANY GRAIN CAN BE SUBSTI-
TUTED, BUT THE TEXTURE OF THE WHEAT BERRY MAKES IT WORTH SEEKING OUT.

4 cups vegetable or chicken broth
1 cup whole-wheat berries,
    soaked overnight and drained
1 cup buckwheat (kasha)
    2 cups frozen peas
1 green bell pepper, seeded and diced
8 scallions, whites only, sliced thin
1/3 cup chopped fresh parsley
1/3 cup lemon juice
1 tablespoon olive oil
1 tablespoon ground cumin
1 teaspoon black pepper
Dash of salt

In a large saucepan bring the broth to a boil. Add the wheat
berries, then reduce heat, cover, and simmer for 40 minutes. Add the
buckwheat and simmer for another 15 to 20 minutes, until all the liq-

THE ANTI-AGING PLAN 201

uid has been absorbed. Remove from the heat and fluff with a fork. Cool.

Meanwhile, prepare the peas according to package instructions. Combine the wheat berries and buckwheat with the peas and all the remaining ingredients in a large bowl. Stir from the bottom up to thoroughly blend in the oil and spices. Adjust the seasonings to taste.

This dish can be prepared a day ahead or allowed to marinate for half an hour. It will survive in warm weather without refrigeration for several hours. It is best marinated overnight in the refrigerator and served slightly chilled.

Calories per serving: 180. Percentage of calories from fat 13%, protein 15%, carbohydrates 72%, 0 mg cholesterol.

❋ Mushroom and Barley Pilaf

Serves 4, makes about 2 2/3 cups

Olive oil cooking spray
2 cups vegetable broth or water
1 small onion, diced
2 cloves garlic, pressed
2 cups sliced fresh mushrooms
1/2 green bell pepper, chopped
1 tablespoon chopped fresh rosemary
   or 2 teaspoons dried
1 tablespoon chopped fresh thyme
   or 2 teaspoons dried
1/2 cup wine
1 cup barley
1 3"strip kombu, soaked 15 minutes and chopped
1 tablespoon chopped fresh dill or 1 teaspoon dried

Spray a large, lidded, flameproof casserole with olive oil. Heat over medium heat. Along with a few tablespoons water or broth, add the onion and garlic. Sauté until the onion begins to turn translucent. Add the mushrooms and bell pepper and sauté for another 2 minutes, adding a little more water if necessary. Stir in the rosemary, thyme and wine. Continue cooking for another 3 minutes. Stir in the barley and sauté a final 3 minutes.

Add the remaining broth or water, the kombu, and dill. Mix thoroughly. Bring to a boil, cover, and place the casserole in the oven. Bake for 30 to 40 minutes, until the barley is tender. Check periodically to see if more liquid is needed.

Serve hot.

Calories per serving: 200. Percentage of calories from fat 3%, protein, 11%, carbohydrates 86%, 0 mg cholesterol.

Pasta

✳ *Macaroni and Cheese*

Serves 8

YES! THE CLASSIC THAT YOUR KIDS WANT IS A 15-MINUTE SIDE DISH (NOT INCLUDING THE 35-MINUTE BAKING TIME). SERVE IT WITH ANY OF THE FOLLOWING: A SIMPLE STIR-FRY, BAKED CHICKEN, OR BEANS AND A SALAD. WE ARE SUGGESTING EXTRA-SHARP CHEDDAR CHEESE BECAUSE THIS BOOSTS THE FLAVOR OF THE ADDED COTTAGE CHEESE AND TOGETHER THEY MAKE A FULL-BODIED FLAVOR THAT CHILDREN LOVE.

THE NOVEL INGREDIENT HERE IS THE WHEAT GERM. WHILE IT DOESN'T CHANGE THE FLAVOR OR TEXTURE OF THE DISH, IT DOES BOOST THE RECOMMENDED DAILY ALLOWANCES FOR VITAMIN E FROM 6% TO 42%, AND VITAMIN K FROM 39% TO 69%.

Olive or canola oil cooking spray
14 ounces whole-wheat
   or brown rice elbow macaroni
1 cup finely chopped onions
1/2 cup finely chopped celery
1/2 teaspoon dried oregano
1/2 teaspoon dried sweet basil
1/4 cup water
1 tablespoon low-sodium soy sauce
4 egg whites
1 1/2 cups low-fat or nonfat cottage cheese
1 1/2 cups evaporated skim milk
1/3 cup wheat germ
1 cup grated extra-sharp low-fat cheddar cheese

Preheat the oven to 350°F. Spray a large baking pan with oil.

Cook the macaroni according to package directions. If using whole wheat, boil for approximately 10 minutes, brown rice pasta slightly longer.

Meanwhile, spray a small skillet with oil. Add the onion and celery, cover, and heat over a medium flame for 3 minutes. Remove cover, add the oregano, basil, and the 1/4 cup water. Cover and cook another 3 minutes. As the liquids evaporate, scrape the rich skillet drippings into the vegetables. Add the soy sauce, cover, and cook another 2 minutes. The vegetables should be slightly crisp.

In a food processor or blender whip the egg whites for 30 seconds. Add the cottage cheese, evaporated skim milk, and wheat germ. Whip 1 minute, just to blend. Add the cooked vegetables and process for a few seconds.

Drain the noodles and place in a large bowl. Stir in the whipped cheese mixture.

Add the macaroni to the prepared baking pan and top with the grated cheddar cheese. Bake for 30 to 40 minutes, until the macaroni is firm and the cheese on top is crusty.

Calories per serving: 360. Percentage of calories from fat 21%, protein 29%, carbohydrates 49%, 12 mg cholesterol.

✳ *Quick Pasta Primavera*

Serves 2

THIS IS SO QUICK AND EASY THAT WE'VE LISTED INGREDIENTS FOR TWO PEOPLE ONLY. IT CAN BE DOUBLED OR HALVED; WE FREQUENTLY WHIP THIS UP WHEN WE'RE EATING ALONE. BE CREATIVE — PRACTICALLY ANY LEFTOVER VEGETABLES IN THE REFRIGERATOR COULD BE ADDED TO THIS. HOWEVER, WE QUITE LIKE THE SIMPLE COMBINATION OF THESE PARTICULAR FLAVORS.

SERVE THIS WITH SIMPLE GREENS AND CREAMY HERB DRESSING AND YOU'LL HAVE AN ELEGANT MEAL IN 20 MINUTES.

1 cup dry whole-wheat spiral or elbow noodles
2/3 cup frozen peas
1 large fresh tomato, chopped
2 tablespoons freshly grated Parmesan cheese
1 clove garlic, pressed
Pinch of chopped fresh parsley
Pinch of chopped fresh basil (optional)
Dash of black pepper (optional)

Bring 4 cups of water to boil in a medium saucepan. Add the noodles and cook for 12 to 15 minutes, according to the package instructions, and depending on the noodles you use.

Meanwhile, cook the peas according to package instructions and drain.

Drain the noodles, and thoroughly mix with the peas and all the remaining ingredients.

Serve hot.

Calories per serving: 282. Percentage of calories from fat 13%, protein 16%, carbohydrates 70%, 8 mg cholesterol.

✳ Creamy Baked Ziti

Serves 8

Italians have truly refined the art of pasta. Here, the shape of the noodle catches creamy ricotta cheese lightly flavored with a hint of marjoram.

We use both the broccoli stalks and flowerets in this dish. Broccoli stalks, which many people throw away, are delicious when properly prepared, with a flavor reminiscent of artichoke hearts.

In a hurry? Skip the egg whites and bake the ziti for only 15 minutes. The egg whites do add protein, and they transform a simple noodle dish into a main meal. Incidentally, egg whites beat up to a greater volume when they are at room temperature. If you are in a hurry, you could take the chill off them by placing them in a small heavy pan and putting it over hot water. Just be careful not to let

THE WHITES COOK.

Olive or canola oil cooking spray
4 bunches broccoli stalks separated from flowerets
1 package (10 ounces) frozen peas
1 pound ziti, elbow macaroni, or shells
4 cloves garlic, pressed
2 large fresh shiitake or
    8 regular mushrooms, coarsely chopped
2 to 3 tablespoons water
1/2 teaspoon marjoram
2 cups low-fat or nonfat ricotta cheese
1 1/2 tablespoons wheat germ
1 cup grated low-fat mozzarella cheese, grated
4 egg whites
Paprika to taste

Preheat the oven to 400°F. Spray a large baking pan with oil.

Prepare the broccoli stalks with a sharp knife by skinning the tough outer layer of stalk. If the stalk inside is fibrous and dry, discard. Chop the broccoli stalks into bite-size pieces and set aside; steam only the broccoli flowerets and set aside.

Cook the peas according to package instructions; drain.

Fill a large saucepan three-fourths full of water and add the pasta. Cook until barely tender, still chewy (before "al dente"). Drain.

While the noodles are cooking, spray a nonstick skillet with oil. Heat over a medium heat and add the garlic. Stir for 3 to 4 minutes, then add the chopped broccoli stalks and shiitake mushrooms. Add a few spoonfuls of water, cover, and cook for 5 minutes. Remove from the heat and stir in the steamed broccoli flowerets.

Stir the marjoram into the ricotta cheese. Arrange one-third of the pasta to cover the bottom of the prepared pan. Spread half of the broccoli over the pasta. Spoon half of the mixture over the broccoli; sprinkle half of the wheat germ over the ricotta. Sprinkle on half the mozzarella. Add another one-third of the pasta, and cover with all of the peas. Spoon on the remaining half of the ricotta and the rest of the wheat germ. Cover the wheat germ with the remaining pasta, then mozzarella.

Beat the egg whites until firm and spread evenly over the casserole. Sprinkle with a little paprika and bake for 20 minutes, or until the top turns golden brown.

Calories per serving: 350. Percentage of calories from fat 19%, protein 24%, carbohydrates 57%, 24 mg cholesterol.

✳ *Pasta Verde*

Serves 4

HOME LATE FROM WORK? WE WHIP UP THIS MEAL EASILY AT THE END OF A LONG DAY. SUNFLOWER SEEDS AND MUSHROOMS PROVIDE TEXTURE WHILE THE COTTAGE CHEESE AND NORI ADD PROTEIN AND B VITAMINS. THIS DISH DOES NOT FREEZE VERY WELL, BUT IT'S SO EASY TO MAKE FRESH. DO USE FRESH BASIL.

    8 ounces whole-wheat fettuccine noodles
    Olive oil cooking spray
    8 fresh mushrooms, stems removed, sliced thin
    4 scallions, whites only, chopped
    2 to 3 tablespoons vegetable broth or water
    3 cups fresh spinach,
        washed and coarsely chopped,
        or 1 package (10 ounces) of frozen spinach, thawed
    2 sheets (each 4" x 2") nori, torn into bite-size pieces
    3 cloves garlic, peeled
    1 cup fresh basil leaves
    1/4 cup grated Parmesan cheese
    3/4 cup low-fat or nonfat cottage cheese
    2 tablespoons grated onion
    1/3 cup sunflower seeds, dry roasted
    Dash each of paprika and black pepper

Cook the noodles according to the package instructions.

Spray a small nonstick skillet with olive oil and heat over a low heat. Add the mushrooms and scallions with a few tablespoons water or broth and dry-fry, stirring frequently, until the mushrooms are thoroughly cooked.

In a medium-size saucepan, steam the spinach for 3 minutes. Add the nori and continue to steam for another minute.

Process the garlic in a food processor until coarsely chopped. With the motor running, add the basil and blend for one minute. Add the cheeses, onion, sunflower seeds and spices. Blend for 1 minute.

Drain the noodles and stir in the spinach, sauce, and the mushrooms. Serve immediately.

Calories per serving: 320. Percentage of calories from fat 22%, protein 24%, carbohydrates 51%, 6 mg cholesterol.

✳ *Thai Noodle Salad*

Serves 8

THE THAIS CALL THIS DISH "PAD THAI." THE RICE NOODLES ARE DELICIOUS, AND WE ESPECIALLY RECOMMEND THEM TO PEOPLE WHO ARE IN THE PROCESS OF CHANGING FROM COMMERCIALLY SOLD PROCESSED AND REFINED NOODLES TO WHOLE-WHEAT NOODLES. THEY ARE LIGHTER THAN WHOLE-WHEAT NOODLES, AND ABSORB SAUCES WELL. YOU CAN FIND THEM IN ASIAN GROCERY STORES AND IN SOME HEALTH FOOD STORES. SOBA NOODLES MAY ALSO BE SUBSTITUTED.

CHICKEN, SHRIMP, OR PORK MAY BE INCLUDED. TRY ANY ONE OR A COMBINATION OF THE THREE. FOLLOW THE DIRECTIONS FOR TOFU, SUBSTITUTING THE MEAT OF YOUR CHOICE.

THIS SALAD'S LOW CALORIC COUNT MEANS THAT YOU MAY EAT TWO SERVINGS. YOU PROBABLY WILL WANT TO ANYWAY! THE FAT COUNT CAN BE REDUCED EVEN MORE BY CUTTING OUT THE PEANUT OIL.

SERVE WITH A SIMPLE SOUP OR GREEN SALAD.

> 12 ounces brown rice noodles
>   or whole-wheat linguine
> 1/3 cup low-sodium soy sauce
> 3 tablespoons almond butter or peanut butter
> 1 tablespoon brown sugar, packed

Olive oil cooking spray
1 whole egg plus 1 egg white, lightly beaten
1 teaspoon peanut oil
4 cloves garlic, minced
8 scallions, white and greens,
    separated and sliced thin
1/4 cup dried hot pepper flakes
2 sheets (each 4" x 2") nori, minced
1 large stalk broccoli, flowerets only
4 large fresh shiitake mushrooms,
    sliced into thin, long strips
6 to 8 ounces firm tofu, cut into 1/4" cubes
2 tablespoons wheat germ
2 cups mung bean sprouts

Cook the noodles according to package instructions. Drain them well, then rinse under cold water. Place them in a bowl with cold water to cover until ready for use. This will prevent them from clumping together.

Combine the soy sauce, nut butter, and brown sugar in a small food processor, or mash with a fork. Set aside.

Spray a small skillet with olive oil. Place the skillet over medium-low heat and add the eggs. Tilt the pan until the eggs cover the bottom of the skillet evenly. When the eggs firm, flip them with a spatula, and cook briefly on the other side. Remove the omelet from the pan and roll up into a long, thin roll on a cutting board. Slice into 1/4-inch pieces and set aside.

Heat the peanut oil in a wok or large skillet. Add the garlic, scallion whites, and pepper. Stir-fry for a minute. Add the nori, broccoli, and shiitake mushrooms, and continue to stir-fry for 5 minutes. Add the tofu, wheat germ, and mung bean sprouts. Cover and cook for 3 minutes, then uncover and stir thoroughly, from the bottom to the top. Add the noodles and the nut butter sauce, stirring to combine everything as evenly as possible with the sauce.

Serve immediately, garnished with rolled egg strips and green scallions. Serve any remaining eggs strips as a side dish.

Calories per serving: 300. Percentage of calories from fat 23%, protein 19%, carbohydrates 58%, 68 mg cholesterol.

Fish

Sesame-Breaded Swordfish
with Mango-Orange Sauce•210
Coriander-Breaded Tuna•212
Herbed Oyster•213
Stovetop-Grilled Salmon•214
Chinese Bouillabaisse •215
Fish Pâté•217

✳ *Sesame-Breaded Swordfish with Mango-Orange Sauce*

Serves 4

THE "BREADING" IN THIS RECIPE IS ACTUALLY FLAVORFUL SESAME SEEDS.
THE FOOD EDITOR OF THE LOS ANGELES TIMES SAID THAT PERHAPS
THE BEST WAY TO EAT A MANGO IS NAKED IN THE SHOWER! SUCH IS ITS REP-
UTATION FOR MESSINESS AND SUCCULENCE.

WHILE INDIA IS THE WORLD'S LARGEST MANGO PRODUCER, MOST OF OUR
MANGOES COME FROM FLORIDA, HAWAII, OR BRAZIL, AND YOU WILL FIND THEM
MAKING THEIR APPEARANCE IN YOUR MARKET EARLIER EVERY YEAR. OR YOU
CAN OFTEN FIND CANNED MANGOES IN THE ASIAN SECTION OF YOUR SUPER-
MARKET. PEARS MAY BE SUBSTITUTED IF MANGOES ARE HARD TO FIND, BUT
USE MANGOES WHENEVER POSSIBLE. THIS SAUCE MAKES FOR A TENDER BAKED
CHICKEN À L'ORANGE AS WELL. SERVE THE STEAKS WITH RICE OR PASTA AND
STEAMED BROCCOLI.

<u>Fish</u>
3 egg whites
1/2 teaspoon low-sodium soy sauce
1/2 cup sesame seeds,
    preferably half white and half black
14 ounces swordfish, halibut,
    or other firm, white fish steaks

<u>Sauce</u>
1 1/2 cups orange juice
2 mangoes, pitted, peeled, and chopped
2 tablespoons peeled
   and minced fresh ginger
2 tablespoons frozen concentrated apple juice
4 scallions, whites only, sliced thinly
12 to 15 large fresh mint leaves, minced
Dash of salt
Pinch of saffron (optional)
2 tablespoons orange liqueur (optional)

Preheat the broiler.

In a 2-quart saucepan bring the 1 1/2 cups orange juice to a gentle simmer. Add all the remaining ingredients and simmer for 15 to 20 minutes, until the sauce has reduced by about one-third. Pour the sauce into a food processor and puree until smooth. If the sauce is too thick, thin with a little orange juice or water. Set aside. Return to the stove to reheat just prior to serving.

Place the egg whites in a shallow bowl and whisk lightly with the soy sauce. Spread the sesame seeds on a plate. Dip each fish steak into the egg whites, and then dredge in the sesame seeds. Broil 10 minutes for a 1" steak.

Calories per serving: 220. Percentage of calories from fat 24%, protein 34%, carbohydrates 42%, 55 mg cholesterol.

✳ *Coriander-Breaded Tuna*

Serves 4

THE "BREADING" HERE IS PURE CRACKED CORIANDER SEEDS AND PEPPER-
CORNS. THIS RECIPE IS SIMPLE, QUICK, AND REALLY UNIQUE. I SERVE IT WITH
RICE PILAF AND A SALAD, OR BROIL IT A LITTLE LONGER AND FLAKE IT FOR DELI-
CIOUS FISH TACOS.

2 egg whites
1/3 cup coriander seeds, cracked
1/4 cup black peppercorns, cracked with the coriander seeds
4 tuna steaks, each about 3 1/2 ounces
Olive oil cooking spray

Lightly beat in the egg whites in a shallow bowl. Spread the coriander seeds and black peppercorns on a plate. Dip each tuna steak into
the egg whites, then dredge the seeds until fully coated.

Spray a large skillet with olive oil and place over high heat. When
the pan is hot, quickly sear the steaks on each side, about 20 seconds.
The tuna is best when it is still pink and tender on the inside, moist on
the outside.

Calories per serving: 145. Percentage of calories from fat 22%, protein 76%, carbohydrates 0, 57 mg cholesterol.

✳ Herbed Oysters

Serves 4

OYSTER LORE FILLS PAGES WITH SUCH ILLUSTRIOUS FANS AS SENECA, NERO, AND LOUIS XIV, WHO COULD CONSUME FIFTY FOR LUNCH. ABRAHAM LINCOLN GAVE OYSTER PARTIES AS WELL.

OYSTERS HAVE BECOME A WEEKLY HABIT FOR US THIS YEAR. THEY ARE VERY LOW IN CALORIES, AND RICH IN ZINC, VITAMIN D, CALCIUM AND IRON, AND ARE ON OUR TOP-20 LIST OF SUPERNUTRITIOUS FOODS. HOWEVER, EAT ONLY OYSTERS THAT HAVE BEEN CULTIVATED IN COLD WATERS.

2 cups water
1 cup millet
1 onion, diced fine
1 pound oysters, shucked fresh or drained canned
1 tablespoon dried sage
1/2 teaspoon ground cumin
2 tablespoons Worcestershire sauce
1 tablespoon bottled chutney
Chopped fresh parsley

In a medium-size saucepan bring two cups of water to a boil. Add the millet and onion. Reduce the heat, cover, and simmer for 20 minutes.

Add the oysters and all the remaining ingredients except the chutney and parsley. Cook another 10 minutes for fresh oysters, 5 minutes for canned.

Remove from the heat and stir, then serve garnished with chutney and parsley.

Calories per serving: 125. Percentage of calories from fat 10%, protein 19%, carbohydrates 42%, 52 mg cholesterol.

✳ *Stovetop-Grilled Salmon*

Serves 4

APART FROM BAKING THE POTATOES, THIS MEAL COOKS UP IN 25 MIN-
UTES, INCLUDING CUTTING TIME. BAKE A FEW EXTRA POTATOES THE DAY
BEFORE AND USE CANNED SALMON TO REALLY SAVE TIME.

THIS SIMPLEST OF WAYS TO PREPARE SALMON SAVES YOU THE CLEANUP OF
BROILING. AND SINCE THE RECIPE NEEDS A FIRMLY COOKED FISH, POACHING
WOULD NOT BE APPROPRIATE.

4 medium-size baking potatoes, scrubbed
Olive oil cooking spray
2 salmon steaks (each about 3 1/2 ounces)
4 cloves garlic, minced
1 onion, coarsely chopped
1 green bell pepper, seeded and coarsely chopped
1 tablespoon black pepper, or to taste
1 teaspoon chopped fresh dill
2 large fresh tomatoes, seeded
    and coarsely chopped
1/4 cup minced fresh parsley

Preheat the oven to 375°F.

Pierce each potato a few times with a fork. Place on a baking sheet
and bake for 1 hour, or until a fork pierces easily into the center of
each. Remove from the oven, cut in half. When cool enough to handle, cut into thick pieces, 1/2" squares.

Spray a large saucepan with olive oil. Lay the salmon steaks side
by side in the pan. Cover and turn the heat on very low. Allow the fish
to simmer in its own juices for 6 to 8 minutes, depending on the thickness of the steaks. A fork should barely be able to flake the meat. As
you will continue cooking this fish with the potatoes, leave it slightly
pink in the middle, still tender. Remove from the heat and use a spatula to lift the steaks out of the pan and set them on a plate. When cool
enough to handle, remove the skin and bones and flake into bite-size
pieces.

Spray a cold large skillet with olive oil, and heat it over a low heat.

Add the garlic and sauté for a few minutes. Now add the onion and bell pepper. Cover and simmer for 3 to 5 minutes, stirring once. Uncover and dry-fry the vegetables, stirring frequently, until the onion browns slightly. Add the potatoes and black pepper and continue to dry-fry, stirring every few minutes. When the potatoes begin to form a crust, add the dill, tomatoes, and the salmon, stirring frequently. Cook for another 5 minutes or longer, until the fish is heated through and there is enough crust to suit you.

Stir in the parsley and serve immediately.

Calories per serving: 325. Percentage of calories from fat 19%, protein 20%, carbohydrates 61%, 16 mg cholesterol.

✳ *Chinese Bouillabaisse*

Serves 8

...OR CHINESE NOODLE SOUP WITH SEAFOOD. WITH THE RECENT POPULARITY OF RAMEN NOODLES, WHOLE-WHEAT OR BUCKWHEAT NOODLES SHOULD BE EASY TO FIND IN YOUR LOCAL MARKET. WHEN SERVED IN THIS MILDLY RED CHILI-LACED BROTH THEY SOAK UP THE SPICES AND TASTE ABSOLUTELY LUSCIOUS.

THIS RECIPE IS SO NUTRITIOUS IT ALMOST QUALIFIES AS A ONE-A-DAY MEGAMEAL. THE SALMON IT CALLS FOR IS AT THE TOP OF THE LIST FOR FISH HIGH IN OMEGA-3 FATTY ACIDS, THE KIND THAT ARE BENEFICIAL FOR COMBATTING HEART DISEASE.

MANY ASIAN MEATS ARE MARINATED PRIOR TO COOKING, AND THIS IS NO EXCEPTION. THE FISH CAN MARINATE WHILE YOU PREPARE THE BROTH AND VEGETABLES. I'VE TAKEN SOME LIBERTIES WITH THE VEGETABLES TO BOOST THE NUTRITIONAL VALUE HERE. BROCCOLI IS NOT OFTEN SERVED IN A FISH-BASED SOUP, BUT IT IS SO HIGH IN SEVERAL VITAMINS THAT EVEN A HALF OF ONE STALK IS WORTH INCLUDING. SERVE WITH A FRESH GREEN SALAD, AND BE SURE TO INCLUDE A NUTCRACKER TO DIG AWAY FOR CRABMEAT.

3 quarts chicken or vegetable broth
1/3 cup mirin (Japanese rice wine) or dry sherry
2 tablespoons low-sodium soy sauce
1 tablespoon molasses
1/4 cup pureed fresh ginger
1 pound salmon fillets,
  sliced crosswise into 1/2" pieces
1 pound medium-size shrimp, shells removed,
  sliced lengthwise into thin slices
4 celery stalks, sliced 1/2" thick on the diagonal
4 cups (2 bunches) diagonally sliced kale
2 leeks, trimmed of greens,
  well washed, and sliced paper thin
2 teaspoons coriander seed
2 teaspoons dried hot pepper flakes
1/2 teaspoon white pepper
1 pound fresh snow peas, ends removed
2 stalks broccoli, flowerets separated from stems,
  stems peeled and cut into 2" x 1/4" strips
2 red bell peppers, seeded and sliced thin
3/4 cup dried arame seaweed
12 ounces whole-wheat noodles
  (ramen or soba noodles)
1 pound crab legs
1 sheet (8" x 7") nori, shredded
1 medium-size cucumber, peeled and sliced thin

In a baking dish, beat 1/4 cup of the broth, the mirin, soy sauce, molasses, and ginger to mix. Add the salmon and shrimp, toss to mix well, and set in the refrigerator.

In a very large kettle bring the remaining broth to a boil. Add the celery, kale, leeks, coriander seeds, hot pepper flakes, and white pepper. Simmer for 10 minutes. Add the snow peas, broccoli, and bell peppers, and continue to simmer another 10 minutes. Add the arame seaweed.

Meanwhile, fill a 2-quart saucepan with water and bring to a boil. Add the noodles and cook for 4 to 6 minutes, according to package instructions. Drain and keep warm.

Add the crab legs to the soup, and simmer for 5 minutes. With a slotted spoon, add the marinated fish and the nori. Simmer for 3 minutes, or until the fish melts in your mouth!

Stir in the noodles.

To serve, ladle a generous portion of noodles, a ladleful of broth, and some vegetables into each bowl. Top with the sliced raw cucumber.

Calories per serving: 436. Percentage of calories from fat 20%, protein 36%, carbohydrates 44%,138 mg cholesterol.

✳ *Fish Pâté*

Serves 4

THE NAME "SARDINE" REFERS TO A NUMBER OF SMALL SEA HERRINGS THAT ARE USUALLY CANNED AND BRINED. THIS METHOD ORIGINATED ON THE ISLAND OF SARDINIA, HENCE, SARDINES.

ONE CAN OF SARDINES PACKED IN TOMATO SAUCE, MUSTARD SAUCE, OR WATER PROVIDES HALF OF YOUR DAILY REQUIREMENT FOR CALCIUM, AND FEATURES ONLY 150 CALORIES. THESE LITTLE FISHES ARE UNSUNG NUTRITIONAL HEROS. THE FOLLOWING PÂTÉ MAKES AN EXCELLENT SANDWICH.

3 cans water-packed sardines
1 tablespoon brewer's yeast
1 teaspoon dijon mustard
3 hard-cooked egg whites
2 scallions, whites only, minced
1 1/2 cups fresh or frozen peas
Minced fresh parsley
Paprika

For Sandwiches
4 pita pockets
2 tomatoes, sliced thin
1/2 onion, sliced thin
4 romaine lettuce leaves

In a food processor puree the sardines. Add the yeast and mustard, then using the pulse mode to blend rather than puree, add the egg whites. Transfer the mixture to a bowl and stir in the scallions.

If using frozen peas, cook according to package directions, drain and cool. If using fresh peas, steam for 6 to 7 minutes, until tender. In a clean food processor bowl, puree the peas.

To serve as a pâté, layer the sardine mixture over the bottom of a small square serving dish. Spread the peas over the sardines. Garnish with a little parsley and paprika.

To serve as sandwiches, open each pita pocket and spread the peas on one side, the sardine mixture on the other, and sandwich the tomato, onion and lettuce between the two.

Calories per 1/2 cup serving of pâté alone: 160. Percentage of calories from fat 30%, protein 42%, carbohydrates 27%, 84 mg cholesterol.

Calories per sandwich: 272. Percentage of calories from fat 18%, protein 30%, carbohydrates 51%, 56 mg cholesterol.

Meat and Poultry

Meat — and we are speaking here first of red meat — is nutrient rich, but its usually high fat content makes a heavy meat diet unhealthy. So if you are a meat eater, choose cuts as low in fat content as possible. For beef there are two things to consider: first, the labeling of cuts from the same part of the animal (Prime cuts have the most fat, Choice cuts come next, and Select grades have the least fat), second, the different locations on the beast. The leanest cuts are those which get the most exercise when the animal moves. These are the neck and shoulder (chuck), lower leg (shank), belly (flank), and upper rear leg (round). Thus, "Select grade top round" steak has the least amount of calories tied up in fat.

If you cook it right, lean meat is just as delicious as fat-marbled meat. Marinating it before cooking will tenderize it. Braising is also a good way to tenderize it. To braise, sear over high heat in a very small amount of oil, then add enough water, broth, or juice to submerge it halfway. Bring the liquid to a boil, cover, and simmer gently on top of the stove for 45 minutes to one hour.

Pork fat is less harmful than beef fat as it contains the essential saturated fatty acid, linoleic acid, whereas beef fat contains mainly the highly saturated palmitic and stearic acids. Veal has lower levels of saturated fat than either pork or beef, which makes it your top choice among red meats. If you buy lunchmeat, choose those labeled "reduced fat content."

Poultry contains less fat than beef, lamb or pork, especially if you remove the skin and visible fat before cooking. Try substituting ground turkey for beef in your hamburger, chili or meatloaf recipes.

While the table below shows us that the caloric content of a standard serving of red meat is not that high, bear in mind that in most of these cuts at least 40 percent of the calories do come from fat. Yet the zinc and iron in red meat are more easily absorbed by the body than the zinc and iron in vegetables. Meat, when prepared properly, is a low-calorie, nutrient-rich food. Glaze meat and poultry with fruit juice concentrate. If using pan drippings, trim off the fat first.

The following table should help you choose a leaner cut of meat. All portions are 31/2 ounce servings, and prepared in accordance with low-fat standards.

Calorie count per 3½ ounce serving

BEEF

Top round	135
Sirloin	133
Flank steak	145
Porterhouse	165
Liver (pan fried)	199
Ground, extra lean	218
Ground, lean	231
Ground, regular	246
Corned	293
Shortribs, lean	295

PORK

Ham, extra lean	193
Canadian bacon	216
Bacon	665

LAMB

Leg, roasted	130
Loin chops, lean	138
Shoulder	148
Ground	263

VEAL

Ground, round	139
Loin chops, lean only	156

CHICKEN

Light meat	117
Dark meat	130
Liver	125

TURKEY

Light meat	114
Dark meat	123
Ground	218

Suggestions

Steaks and chops
Cook quickly over high heat, broil, or barbecue.

Beef: flank or chuck steak, top round, sirloin and fat-trimmed tenderloin, bottom round; avoid rib, club, shoulder, brisket and T-bone steaks.

Lamb: Loin chops, shanks; avoid rib chops, shoulder.

Pork: Canadian bacon, center-cut pork chop, loin cutlets, cured ham, fat-trimmed rump; avoid rib chops, spareribs, bacon, shoulder, hock, feet.

Roasts
Use dry heat oven roasting.

Beef: Fat trimmed tenderloin, top round, eye of round, rump, sirloin; avoid rib roasts.

Lamb: Fat trimmed leg of lamb; avoid rib, loin, shoulder.

Pork: Fat trimmed ham, tenderloin, center-cut loin; avoid shoulder and fat marbled roasts.

Stews, pot roasts
Cook slowly, allow meat to simmer in liquids.

Beef: flank, fat trimmed bottom round, chuck steak; avoid shoulder, short ribs, brisket.

Lamb: shank; avoid shoulder

Pork: Fat trimmed rump, cured ham; avoid shoulder, ribs, hock, feet.

The recipes are examples of how traditional recipes can be adapted to the Anti-Aging Plan. Using a lean cut of meat and a vegetable based sauce or, using meat as an ingredient equal to a vegetable in a larger recipe, as we do in our One-A-Day Megameals and Free-Choice recipes, are healthier ways to go.

Peppered Steak•222
Best Hamburgers•223
Best Meatballs in Tomato Sauce•224

✳ *Peppered Steak*

Serves 4

WE RECOMMEND THAT YOU RETHINK THE ROLE OF MEAT AT YOUR MEALS. AMERICANS AND EUROPEANS TEND TO SEE IT AS THE MAIN EVENT OF A MEAL, AND THEREFORE CONSUME IT IN LARGE QUANTITIES. YOU WILL FEEL BETTER, MORE ALERT, LIGHTER, IF YOU SEE MEAT AS SOMETHING TO USE IN SMALLER QUANTITIES, ONE OF MANY INGREDIENTS IN A LARGER RECIPE. THIS IS EASY TO DO IN STIR-FRIES, CASSEROLES, AND STEWS, IN WHICH YOU SIMPLY DECREASE THE TRADITIONAL AMOUNT OF MEAT AND INCREASE THE QUANTITY OF ALL OF THE OTHER INGREDIENTS. YET EVEN WHEN YOU COME TO A RECIPE SUCH AS THIS, YOU CAN STILL DO AT LEAST TWO THINGS TO LIGHTEN UP YOUR MEAL: (1) CONSUME, AS YOUR NORMAL PORTION OF MEAT, NO MORE THAN 31/2 OUNCES, (WHICH IS THE PORTION SIZE RECOMMENDED BY THE FOOD AND NUTRITION BOARD OF THE FEDERAL GOVERNMENT) AND (2) SURROUND IT ON YOUR PLATE WITH PLENTY OF LOW-FAT GRAINS, VEGETABLES, OR SAUCES. USE A LEAN CUT OF BEEF, SUCH AS TOP ROUND, SIRLOIN, OR FLANK STEAK. TRIM OFF AS MUCH FAT AS POSSIBLE, AND CAREFULLY MONITOR COOKING TIME. WITH A LEAN CUT OF MEAT, OVERCOOKING WILL YIELD A DRY STEAK.

PROPERLY PREPARED, THIS LEAN STEAK IS GREAT. AND MAKES A WONDERFUL SANDWICH.

Sprinkle both sides of one 14-ounce top round, sirloin, or flank steak with coarsely ground black pepper. Press the pepper into the steak with a rolling pin or large spoon. Press in well.

Broil or barbecue until done to your liking (not more than 10 minutes total for medium well). Make a small cut into the meat to check for doneness.

Calories per serving: 135. Percent of calories from: fat 33%, protein 66%, carbohydrate 0%, 51 mg cholesterol.

✳ *Best Hamburgers*

Serves 4

BARBECUE SEASON LASTS A LONG TIME IN SOUTHERN CALIFORNIA. HERE IS A CREATIVE WAY TO FORTIFY HAMBURGERS NUTRITIONALLY AND CUT DOWN ON THE AMOUNT OF MEAT.

NUTRITIONALLY, BEEF IS A FATTIER PROTEIN THAN TURKEY BUT IT ALSO HAS TWICE AS MUCH IRON. TURKEY HAS NO VITAMIN B12, BUT THE BRAN FLAKES INCLUDED HERE CARRY TWICE AS MUCH IRON AS THE BEEF, AND ARE AS HIGH IN B12, SO THE TURKEY FORTIFIED WITH THE BRAN FLAKES IN THIS RECIPE IS AN EXCELLENT ALTERNATIVE TO BEEF.

DOUBLE THE RECIPE AND FREEZE HALF FOR BEST MEATBALLS IN TOMATO SAUCE.

1/2 large sweet potato
1/2 cup finely chopped onion
1/4 cup finely chopped green bell pepper
3/4 cup bran flakes or wheat bran
1/4 cup wheat germ
2 cloves garlic, pressed
1 teaspoon dried oregano
1 teaspoon dried basil
Dash each of pepper and salt (optional)
8 ounces extra-lean ground beef or turkey
Olive oil cooking spray
Whole-wheat hamburger buns or pita pockets

In a food processor finely grate the sweet potato and set aside in a large bowl. Chop the onion and pepper in the food processor and add to the sweet potato along with the bran flakes, wheat germ, garlic, herbs, and seasonings.

Mix thoroughly with meat and form 4 large patties. Your bare hands make the best mixers.

Spray a large skillet with olive oil and fry the patties over medium heat until cooked to your liking. Or broil, or barbecue.

Serve in hamburger buns or pita pockets.

In the hamburger, using extra-lean ground beef: Calories per patty: 200. Percent of calories from fat 34%, protein 28%, carbohydrates 37%, 41 mg cholesterol.

In the hamburger, using ground flank steak: Calories per patty: 170. Percent of calories from fat 23%, protein 39%, carbohydrates 38%, 33 mg cholesterol.

In the turkeyburger, using commercial ground turkey: Calories per patty: 203. Percent of calories from fat 34%, protein, 34%, carbohydrates 39%, 38 mg cholesterol.

In the turkeyburger, using ground white meat, no skin: Calories per patty: 165. Percent of calories from fat 14%, protein 46%, carbohydrates 39%, 38 mg cholesterol.

✳ Best Meatballs with Tomato Sauce

Serves 4, makes about 20

THE MIXTURE USED IN THE BEST HAMBURGERS RECIPE EASILY ADAPTS TO THESE MEATBALLS. THEY ARE DELICIOUS EITHER HOT OVER WHOLE-WHEAT PASTA WITH NO-FAT CANNED OR HOMEMADE TOMATO SAUCE; OR SERVE IN A WHOLE WHEAT PITA POCKET WITH SHREDDED LETTUCE AND SLICED TOMATO. DOUBLE THE QUANTITY OF THE MEAT MIXTURE AND FREEZE SOME FOR BEST HAMBURGERS.

Meat mixture from Best Hamburgers
Sauce
Olive oil cooking spray
1 large onion, minced
4 cloves garlic, minced
8 large plum tomatoes or 4 medium-size
    beefsteak tomatoes, peeled and seeded
    then coarsely chopped
1/2 green bell pepper, chopped into bite-size pieces
1 tablespoon dried oregano
1 teaspoon paprika
1/2 teaspoon rosemary

Preheat the oven to 350°F.

Prepare the meat mixture and set aside.

For the sauce, spray a medium nonstick saucepan with olive oil and heat over a low flame. Sauté the onions and garlic until the onion is translucent and soft. Add the tomatoes, bell pepper, and herbs. Simmer, covered, for 45 minutes. Uncover and simmer an additional 20 minutes to thicken. Using a rounded soup spoon, shape the meat mixture into 1" meatballs.

Spoon 1/4 cup of the sauce into the bottom of a large baking dish. Arrange the meatballs into two layers. Spoon the rest of the sauce over all and bake for 35 minutes.

Calories per meatball using extra-lean ground beef: 40. Percent of calories from fat 34%, protein 28%, carbohydrates 37%, 8 mg cholesterol.

Calories per meatball using ground flank steak: 34. Percent of calories from fat 23%, protein 39%, carbohydrates 38%, 6 mg cholesterol.

Calories per turkeyball using commercial ground turkey: 40. Percent of calories from fat 34%, protein 34%, carbohydrates 39%, 7 mg cholesterol.

Calories per turkeyball, using ground white meat, no skin: 33. Percent of calories from fat 14%, protein 46%, carbohydrates 39%, 6 mg cholesterol.

✳ Chicken Fajitas with Salsa

Serves 8

Fᴀᴊɪᴛᴀs ᴀʀᴇ ᴇxᴛʀᴇᴍᴇʟʏ ᴘᴏᴘᴜʟᴀʀ ɪɴ Lᴏs Aɴɢᴇʟᴇs. Oғᴛᴇɴ ᴘʀᴇᴘᴀʀᴇᴅ ᴡɪᴛʜ ʙᴇᴇғ, I'ᴠᴇ ɪɴᴄʟᴜᴅᴇᴅ ᴛʜᴇᴍ ʜᴇʀᴇ ᴡɪᴛʜ ᴄʜɪᴄᴋᴇɴ ᴏʀ ᴛᴜʀᴋᴇʏ. Fᴀᴊɪᴛᴀs ᴀʀᴇ ᴜsᴜᴀʟʟʏ ᴡʀᴀᴘᴘᴇᴅ ɪɴ ᴀ ᴛᴏʀᴛɪʟʟᴀ ᴀɴᴅ sᴇʀᴠᴇᴅ ᴡɪᴛʜ sᴀʟsᴀ. Tʜᴇʏ ᴀʀᴇ ᴠᴇʀʏ ᴇᴀsʏ ᴛᴏ ᴘʀᴇᴘᴀʀᴇ, ᴀɴᴅ ᴄᴀɴ ʙᴇ ʙᴀʀʙᴇᴄᴜᴇᴅ ᴏʀ ʙʀᴏɪʟᴇᴅ ᴀs ᴇᴀsɪʟʏ ᴀs ᴅʀʏ-ғʀɪᴇᴅ ɪɴ ᴀ ᴘᴀɴ.

Tʜᴇ sᴇᴄʀᴇᴛ ᴛᴏ ᴀ ɢᴏᴏᴅ sᴀʟsᴀ ɪs ғʀᴇsʜ ɪɴɢʀᴇᴅɪᴇɴᴛs. Iᴛ ʀᴇᴀʟʟʏ ᴍᴀᴋᴇs ᴀ ᴅɪғғᴇʀᴇɴᴄᴇ. Tʜɪs ɪs ᴀ ᴠᴇʀʏ ʙᴀsɪᴄ ᴀɴᴅ sɪᴍᴘʟᴇ sᴀʟsᴀ. Fʀᴇsʜ ɪɴɢʀᴇᴅɪᴇɴᴛs, ɪᴛ ɴᴇᴇᴅs ɴᴏᴛʜɪɴɢ ᴇʟsᴇ.

<u>Marinade</u>
Juice of 4 large oranges
Juice of 6 limes
1/4 cup red wine vinegar
1 teaspoon olive oil
8 cloves garlic, minced
4 to 6 teaspoons dried hot pepper flakes
2 teaspoons dried oregano, crushed
1/4 cup fresh cilantro, chopped

<u>Fajitas</u>
2 pounds skinless, boneless chicken breasts,
    sliced into bite-size pieces
2 onions, halved and sliced very thin

2 large red peppers, seeded and sliced into thin strips
2 large green peppers, seeded and sliced into thin strips

8 corn tortillas or whole-wheat chapatis

Salsa
6 large fresh tomatoes, diced
2 red onions, chopped fine
1 yellow onion, chopped fine
1 cup chopped fresh cilantro
2 fresh jalapeño chiles, seeded and minced
1 cup frozen corn kernels,
    cooked according to package directions,
    or fresh, steamed and cut from the cob.

Mix together all of the ingredients for the marinade and place in a baking pan or casserole dish. Add the chicken. Marinade for a minimum of 2 hours, preferably overnight.

For salsa, mix all ingredients together and refrigerate for 1 hour.

There are three ways to cook a succulent serving of fajitas. You may choose to barbecue, broil or dry-fry.

To barbecue: Use a special barbecue screen placed over the coals, because the pepper slices are too thin to thread onto a skewer. These fajitas will cook quickly, so turn them as soon as they begin to blacken.

To broil: Broiling is similar. Pour the chicken and its marinade and peppers into a shallow baking pan. Add the peppers and onions and place under a preheated broiler for 4 to 5 minutes, or until the chicken blackens slightly. Remove from the heat and stir. Return to the broiler and cook for an additional 2 minutes.

To dry-fry: Spray a large skillet with nonstick olive oil. Add the onions. Dry-fry over medium heat, stirring frequently for 5 minutes, or until the onions turn translucent. Add the peppers and a little of the chicken marinade. Simmer for 5 to 7 minutes, until the peppers have softened. Remove the peppers and onions to a dish. Remove the skillet from the heat, wipe out, and let cool before spraying again with olive oil. Return the skillet to the heat and quickly sear the chicken. Reduce heat and add all the marinade, the peppers, and onions.

Simmer for 6 to 10 minutes, depending on the thickness of the chicken pieces.

To serve, heat the tortillas by steaming them in a double boiler or spraying them with a little water, wrapping in foil, and heating in the oven for 5 minutes. Fill each tortilla with one eighth of the chicken and 2 tablespoons of salsa. They will be filled to the brim!

Calories per serving (fajitas): 290. Percentage of calories from fat 10%, protein 60%, carbohydrates 30%, 74 mg cholesterol.

Calories per 2 large tablespoons of salsa: 45. Percentage of calories from fat 6%, protein 14%, carbohydrates 80%, 0 cholesterol.

☀ *Teriyaki Chicken*

Serves 8

As with the Chicken Fajitas, this dish cooks up in minutes. If possible, marinate the chicken overnight. Broiling is my favorite way of preparing this because the vegetable juices combine with the marinade and make a wonderful sauce. Teriyaki chicken can be barbecued, but you will lose those wonderful vegetable drippings.

Serve with simple rice, a vegetable rice pilaf, or noodles.

Marinade
1 cup mirin(Japanese rice wine) or dry sherry
1 cup low-sodium soy sauce or
     Bragg's Liquid Aminos
1 cup chicken or vegetable broth, or water
1/4 cup fresh peeled and grated ginger
8 cloves garlic, minced
1/4 cup honey
1 teaspoon sesame oil

Chicken and Vegetables
2 pounds skinless, boneless chicken breast,
     sliced into bite-size pieces

2 large green bell peppers, cut into 1" squares
4 large onions, quartered
2 pounds fresh mushrooms, stemmed and halved
16 cherry tomatoes

Preheat the broiler.

Transfer the chicken and marinade to a large broiler pan and add all the vegetables. Broil for 7 to 8 minutes, or until the onions and chicken are charred on the edges only. Remove from broiler, stir, then return to the broiler and cook for an additional 4 to 5 minutes.

Calories per serving: 220. Percentage of calories from fat 13%, protein 70%, carbohydrates 17%, 73 mg cholesterol.

✳ Baked Chicken in Pear Sauce

Serves 4

THIS PEAR SAUCE COMPLEMENTS FISH AS WELL AS POULTRY. SERVE THIS WITH COUSCOUS WITH PEAS AND MINT, WITH THE CURRIED TWO-GRAIN SALAD, SIMPLE RICE, BARLEY, OR ANY OTHER GRAIN.

1 1/2 cups orange juice
2 fresh ripe pears, peeled, cored and chopped
1 tablespoon peeled and minced fresh ginger
2 tablespoons frozen apple juice concentrate
4 scallions, whites only, sliced thinly
12 to 15 large fresh mint leaves, minced
Dash of salt
Pinch of saffron
2 large skinless, boneless chicken breasts

Preheat the oven to 350°F.

In a small saucepan, bring the orange juice to a gentle simmer. Add the pears, ginger, apple juice concentrate, scallions, mint, salt, and saffron and simmer for 15 to 20 minutes, until the sauce has reduced by one-third. Puree the mixture in a food processor until smooth.

Spoon a few tablespoons of sauce into a square baking pan. Place the chicken breasts in the pan skinned-side down and cover with the remaining sauce. Cover the pan with aluminum foil and bake for 20 minutes covered. Remove foil and bake another 10 minutes. Remove the chicken breasts and set aside; keep warm. Whisk or puree the sauce with the chicken drippings and spoon over the chicken. Serve any remaining sauce on the side.

Calories per serving: 220. Percentage of calories from fat 90%, protein 69%, carbohydrates 22%, 73 mg cholesterol.

✳ Chinese Chicken with Broccoli and Cashews

Serves 8

THIS DISH, CALLED KUNG PAO, CAN BE WHIPPED UP IN 30 MINUTES AND SERVED OVER RICE OR PASTA, WITH A SIMPLE GREEN SALAD ON THE SIDE. TO REDUCE THE FAT INTAKE SIGNIFICANTLY, OMIT THE CASHEWS.

    4 skinless boneless chicken breasts,
        cut into 1/2" cubes
    1/4 cup water
    1 tablespoon dry sherry
    2 tablespoons low-sodium soy sauce
    1/4 cup dry white wine
    1 tablespoon cornstarch
    1/2 teaspoon honey
    1 teaspoon rice vinegar
    Olive oil cooking spray
    8 whole dried red peppers, or
        1/3 teaspoon hot pepper flakes
    8 scallions, whites only, chopped
    3 cloves garlic, minced
    1 tablespoon peeled and minced fresh ginger
    4 cups small broccoli flowerets
    1/4 cup cashew nut pieces, toasted

Combine the water, sherry, and 1 tablespoon of the soy sauce in a bowl. Add the chicken pieces and marinate for 10 minutes.

Combine the wine, remaining tablespoon soy sauce, cornstarch, honey, and vinegar in a small bowl and beat to blend. Set the sauce within easy reach of the stove.

Spray a large skillet with olive oil. Heat over a medium heat for 30 seconds. Stir-fry the red peppers or pepper flakes for 2 minutes. Add the chicken and cook until almost done, about 4 minutes. Stir frequently, separating the chicken pieces. Remove the chicken and red peppers with a slotted spoon. Discard the peppers.

Add the scallions, garlic, and ginger and stir-fry for 1 minute. Add the broccoli, cover, and cook for 2 minutes. Remove the cover and re-add the chicken. Stir thoroughly.

Slowly, in a thin stream, pour the sauce evenly into the skillet while stirring constantly. Cover and simmer for 3 minutes. When the sauce has thickened, add the cashews.

Calories per serving: 293. Percentage of calories from fat 23%, protein 47%, carbohydrates 35%, 73 mg cholesterol.

☀ Roasted Chicken with Bordelaise Sauce

Serves 5

FOR YEARS WE HAVE BEEN REMOVING THE SKIN OF CHICKEN PRIOR TO BAKING TO REDUCE THE FAT CONTENT. THE LATEST RESEARCH INDICATES THAT AS LONG AS THE SKIN IS NOT CONSUMED, REMOVING IT BEFORE OR AFTER COOKING WILL NOT ALTER THE FAT CONTENT. THIS REDUCES YOUR PREPARATION TIME CONSIDERABLY.

THE DRY HEAT OF ROASTING IS ONE OF THE EASIEST WAYS TO PREPARE POULTRY.

    1 large roasting chicken or
        2 small chickens (about 6 pounds total)
    2 cups chicken broth
    1 teaspoon molasses

2 teaspoons tomato paste
1 bay leaf
1/2 teaspoon dried oregano, crushed
1 teaspoon dried thyme, crushed
1 teaspoon dried rosemary
1/2 cup dry red wine
3 tablespoons cornstarch

Preheat oven to 425°F.

Place the bird or birds breast-side up on a roasting rack in a large roasting pan. With a large bird, roast for 30 minutes prior to turning; smaller birds will vary depending on size. Turn the chickens over and continue to roast for another 30 to 45 minutes, for a total roasting time of 50 to 75 minutes. To test for doneness, gently press a knife into a breast. No pink juices should flow. While the spearing method is the best to assure that your meat is done, you can also test the bird by wiggling a drumstick. It should be quite free and loose.

Transfer the chicken to a platter and let stand while you prepare the sauce.

Heat the broth in a medium-size saucepan. Add the molasses, tomato paste, bay leaf, oregano, thyme, and rosemary, stirring to blend. Bring slowly to a simmering boil. Stir constantly to blend in the tomato paste. Mix the wine into the cornstarch. Using a wire whisk, add slowly to the saucepan. Heat and stir a few minutes, until the sauce thickens. Serve alongside the chicken.

Calories per serving: 140 (light meat), 170 (dark meat). Percentage of calories in light meat from fat 11%, protein 71%, carbohydrates 15%, 213 mg cholesterol; in dark meat from fat 27%, protein 58%, carbohydrates 14%, 213 mg cholesterol. Sauce: Calories per 1/2 cup serving: 30. Percentage of calories from fat 20%, protein 33%, carbohydrates 46%, 0 mg cholesterol.

❋ Poultry Loaf with Stroganoff Sauce

Serves 8

THERE'S NOTHING QUITE AS TRADITIONAL AND CONVENIENT AS MEATLOAF!
SERVED ELEGANTLY WITH OUR STROGANOFF SAUCE OR SIMPLY AS A SANDWICH,
THIS LOW-FAT POULTRY LOAF WILL BE "GOBBLED" UP IN NO TIME. SERVE WITH
STEAMED BROCCOLI.

1 cup bulgur wheat
2 cups boiling water
Canola oil cooking spray
2 russet potatoes, sliced into 1/4" pieces
Black pepper
1 package frozen (10 ounces) chopped spinach
2 pounds ground turkey or chicken
1/2 cup wheat bran flakes
1/2 cup wheat germ
4 egg whites
2 medium-size onions, diced fine
1 large green bell pepper, seeded and chopped fine
3 sheets nori (each 4" x 2"),
    chopped fine in a food processor
1/3 cup ketchup
2 tablespoon prepared mustard

Preheat the oven to 350°F.
Soak the bulgur in the 2 cups of water for 15 minutes.
Meanwhile, spray a non-stick cookie sheet with canola oil. Arrange
the potato slices on the sheet in one layer and sprinkle with black pepper. Bake the potato slices for 15 minutes, or until softened but
not dry.
Cook the spinach according to package instructions. Drain the
spinach well, then press excess liquid out with a spoon.
Drain the bulgur thoroughly and place in a large bowl. Add the
turkey with bran flakes, wheat germ, egg whites, onions, bell pepper,
nori, ketchup, and mustard. Use your hands to thoroughly blend
everything together.

Line the bottom of two 9" x 5" x 3" loaf pans with half of the cooked spinach. Take one-fourth of the turkey for each pan and press it firmly over the spinach. Arrange half of the baked potatoes over the turkey, then the remaining turkey.

Bake the loaves for 45 minutes to an hour. The turkey will turn tough and dry if overdone. A knife inserted into the center of the loaf should draw clear juices bubbling to the surface. If no juices bubble, remove immediately. If the juices are pinkish, bake a little longer. Cool for 10 minutes before serving, accompanied, if desired, by the following sauce.

Stroganoff sauce
3/4 cup nonfat dry milk
2 cups nonfat (skim) milk
1/3 cup soybean flour or whole-wheat flour
2 cups fresh mushrooms, quartered
1/2 teaspoon low-sodium soy sauce
1/2 teaspoon dried tarragon
1/4 teaspoon ground sage

Spray a medium-size skillet with olive oil. Heat over a low heat and add the mushrooms. Stir-fry until the mushrooms are soft. Drizzle in a little low-sodium soy sauce. Set aside.

Heat 1 cup of the skim milk in a medium-size saucepan until warm; do not scald. Slowly sift in the flour, whisking constantly to blend and avoid lumps. Add the nonfat dry milk gradually, stirring constantly and slowly. Pour in the remaining skim milk. Continue to stir. When thoroughly heated, add the braised mushrooms and the herbs.

Serve with Poultry Loaf or over grains.

Calories per serving with Stroganoff sauce: 549. Percentage of calories from fat 20%, protein 35%, carbohydrates 45%, 76 mg cholesterol.

Salads

❋ Asparagus Guacamole

Serves 6

THIS RECIPE IS LIGHTER THAN ITS AVOCADO NAMESAKE, AND DELICIOUSLY CREAMY. SERVE WITH BAKED (NOT FRIED) CORN TORTILLAS, WHICH ARE NOW COMMERCIALLY AVAILABLE, OR BAKE YOUR OWN (SEE BELOW). OR USE IT AS A SIDE DISH ALONG WITH BROILED MEATS, OR AS A SANDWICH FILLING. FOR A SAVORY SALAD DRESSING, MIX WITH NONFAT YOGURT TO TASTE.

8 fresh asparagus spears
1/2 cup low-fat or nonfat cottage cheese
     or soft tofu
1 clove garlic
Juice of 1/2 lemon
Salsa, bottled or homemade to taste

Steam the asparagus until tender, about 5 minutes. Plunge briefly into ice water to retain its bright green color. Be sure to do this; the colorfulness of the guacamole will enhance your enjoyment of it.

In a food processor, with the blade running, add the garlic first, the asparagus, and then cottage cheese or tofu. Process the mixture until the cottage cheese's curds have totally disappeared and the consistency is velvety smooth. Stir in the lemon juice and salsa.

Note: You can also prepare this with broccoli stems (no flowerets), substituting 8 stems for the asparagus. Trim off any leaves and peel the thick outer skin off each. Steam till stems are totally tender, from 20 to 30 minutes depending on thickness. Put the stems in the food processor and process until they are velvety smooth before adding the other ingredients.

Calories per serving: 40. Percent of calories from fat 9%, protein 48%, carbohydrates 43%, 1 mg cholesterol.

✳ *Baked Tortilla Chips*

Makes 80 chips

8 soft corn tortillas (not pre-fried)
Salt in moderation
Seasonings

Heat the oven to 200°F.

Cut each of 8 soft tortillas into 10 wedges as you would a pizza and arrange on a large cookie sheet so they do not overlap. Sprinkle with the seasonings of your choice (salt, mild or hot chili powder, cayenne pepper, cumin, black pepper, dried hot pepper flakes, onion powder, garlic powder, etc.) to taste. Bake 30 to 45 minutes, or until crisp.

Calories per serving: 84. Percent of calories from fat 14%, protein 12%, carbohydrates 74%, 1 mg cholesterol.

❋ Mixed Greens with Poppy Seed Dressing

Serves 4

THE STRONG FLAVORS OF THESE GREENS COMPLEMENT THIS SLIGHTLY SWEET SALAD DRESSING. ENDIVE IS SLIGHTLY BITTER WHILE WATERCRESS HAS A SHARP, FRESH SNAP TO IT. IF THESE ARE DIFFICULT TO FIND, SUBSTITUTE ANY GREEN LEAFY LETTUCE. SERVED ALONG WITH PASTA, FISH OR POULTRY, THIS SALAD REMINDS YOU THAT VEGETABLES ARE AS INTOXICATINGLY DELICIOUS AND SATISFYING AS THE RICHEST OF FOODS. THE DRESSING MAKES ALMOST 1 CUP, ENOUGH FOR 12 SERVINGS. REFRIGERATE UNUSED DRESSINGS IN A TIGHTLY CAPPED JAR, UP TO 7 DAYS.

Salad
1 head butter lettuce
1/2 head curly endive
1 bunch watercress
1/2 medium peeled daikon
    or 4 red radishes, sliced very thin
1/2 ripe avocado, peeled, seeded, and diced fine
5 whole scallions, sliced thin
4 fresh mint leaves (optional but
    strongly recommended)

Dressing
1/3 cup honey
1/4 cup vegetable broth
3 tablespoons rice or balsamic vinegar
2 tablespoons poppy seeds
1 1/2 tablespoons lemon juice
1 tablespoon prepared mustard
1 teaspoon low-sodium soy sauce

Wash and thoroughly drain all the greens. Use a salad spinner to remove any excess water or pat the greens dry. The dryness of the greens is essential. (Some of the world's top caterers spread out their greens and turn an electric fan on them to dry them!)

Tear the greens into bite-size pieces and mix them all together in a large bowl. Add the avocado, daikon or radish and scallions. Mix lightly and set aside.

Mix all the ingredients for the dressing in a jar, cap tightly and shake. Add one third of the dressing to the salad and blend lightly, stirring from the bottom to the top.

Garnish each serving with a mint leaf.

Serve chilled.

Calories per serving (with 1 tablespoon dressing): 100. Percent of calories from fat 24%, protein 5%, carbohydrates 70%, 2 mg cholesterol.

✳ *Simple Greens with Creamy Herb Dressing*

Serves 4

THIS IS A REALLY SIMPLE YET GOURMET SIDE DISH. IF YOUR GROCERY CARRIES THEM, MIXED BABY GREENS BY THE POUND OR PREPACKAGED WILL SAVE YOU TIME. TO EXPAND THIS INTO A FULL LUNCH SALAD SIMPLY ADD SOME AVOCADO AND SUNFLOWER SEEDS; TO REDUCE THE FAT INTAKE BY 50 PERCENT, USE CHOPPED EGG WHITES ONLY. IF YOU CANNOT FIND WATERCRESS OR RADICCHIO, TRY NAPA CABBAGE AND ITALIAN PARSLEY.

Salad
1 small head butter lettuce
1 bunch fresh spinach
1 bunch watercress
1 small head radicchio
1/2 cup fresh cilantro leaves
4 whole scallions, chopped
2 medium-size carrots, grated
1 cup frozen peas, cooked and drained
2 hard-cooked eggs, chopped
1 tablespoon grated Parmesan cheese

Dressing
1/2 cup nonfat yogurt
1 clove fresh garlic, minced
1/2 teaspoon black pepper
1/2 teaspoon marjoram
1/2 teaspoon dill (optional)

Wash, drain, and thoroughly dry all the greens, then tear or chop into bite-size pieces. Place in a large bowl and add the vegetables, eggs, and cheese together. Toss lightly.

In a separate bowl blend the dressing. Add to the salad just before serving.

Calories per serving: 90. Percent of calories from fat 21%, protein 34%, carbohydrates 44%, 5 mg cholesterol.

✳ Beans-and-Greens Salad

Serves 4

THE GRATED CHEESE IN THIS SALAD GIVES IT A CREAMY TEXTURE. SERVE WITH ORANGE VEGETABLE SOUP OR A SIDE DISH OF ROASTED POTATOES.

1 head butter or romaine lettuce
3/4 cup canned garbanzo beans (chickpeas)
3/4 cup canned black beans
1 cup shredded bok choy, both leaves and stems
1/3 cup grated low-fat or nonfat cheddar
    or Monterey Jack cheese
1/2 teaspoon olive oil
2 tablespoons lemon juice
1 tablespoon tarragon vinegar

Wash, drain, and tear the lettuce into bite-size pieces. Place in a bowl and mix in the beans, bok choy, and cheese.

In a small bowl beat the oil, lemon juice, and vinegar. Add to the salad and toss lightly.

Calories per serving: 112. Percent of calories from fat 33%, protein 23%, carbohydrates 44%, 12 mg cholesterol.

❋ *Vegetable Smorgasbord Salad*

Serves 4

WE PREPARE THIS SPECIAL SALAD IN QUANTITY, BECAUSE IT REMAINS BEAUTIFULLY FRESH IN THE REFRIGERATOR FOR 2 TO 3 DAYS. REFRIGERATE WITHOUT THE LETTUCE LEAVES: THE LETTUCE MUST ALWAYS BE ADDED FRESH AT THE LAST MINUTE, JUST BEFORE SERVING. SERVED WITH GOOD, FRESH WHOLE-WHEAT BREAD, THIS SALAD IS CRUNCHY, SWEET, SPICY, AND INCREDIBLY SATISFYING. IT'S ONE OF OUR FAVORITES.

Salad
  1/3 cup garbanzo beans (chickpeas),
      soaked overnight and drained
  1/2 cup cowpeas(black-eyed peas),
      soaked with the garbanzo beans
  1/3 cup brown rice
  1/4 cup wild rice
  1/3 cup bran flakes
  1 small sweet potato, quartered
  2 carrots, sliced into 1/2" rounds
  1 broccoli stalk, (flowerets separated),
      stem chopped into bite-size pieces
  6 fresh mushrooms, sliced
  1 fresh tomato, chopped
  1 medium-size red or green bell pepper,
      seeded and sliced into thin strips
  1 small summer squash, halved lengthwise and sliced
  1 small onion, sliced thin
  1/2 cup shredded red cabbage
  1/2 cup chopped fresh parsley
  1/2 cup raisins (optional)

Dressing
3/4 cup plain yogurt
1/2 cup buttermilk
1/3 cup balsamic vinegar
Dried herbs of choice: marjoram/dill, tarragon/basil, etc.
Black pepper to taste

6 leaves romaine lettuce, washed, drained,
     dried, and torn into bite-size pieces

Place the drained beans in a small pot and add water to cover. Over medium flame, bring to a boil, reduce the heat, simmer and cover for 30 to 40 minutes.

Fill another small pot with 1 1/2 cups water. Bring to a boil. Add the brown and wild rice, cover, reduce the heat, and simmer for 45 minutes. Stir in the bran flakes during the last 5 minutes of cooking.

Meanwhile, steam the sweet potato for 15 to 20 minutes, adding the carrots after the first 5 minutes and the broccoli after another 5 minutes. The vegetables should be tender but crisp. When cool enough to handle, cut potatoes into thick, chunky pieces.

Drain the beans and cool under cold running water. Fluff the rice to allow it to cool, and to prevent clumps.

In a large bowl combine the sliced mushrooms, tomato, bell pepper, squash, onion, cabbage, and the steamed vegetables. Mix in the beans, rice, parsley and raisins. In a separate bowl, blend the dressing ingredients together with a wire whisk. Add to the salad. Note: Hands work best to mix in the dressing.

Add the lettuce just prior to serving.

Calories per serving: 460. Percent of calories from fat 8%, protein 21%, carbohydrates 71%, 5 mg cholesterol.

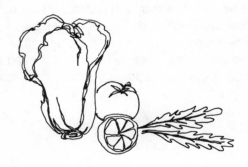

✳ *Marinated Six-Vegetable Salad*

Serves 12

THIS MARINATED, COOKED SALAD MAKES A WONDERFUL FEATURE FOR A
BABY SHOWER OR FOR LUNCH GUESTS. THE POTATOES AND COTTAGE CHEESE
GIVE PROTEIN AND A CREAMY TEXTURE. WE LOVE THIS SALAD WITH WHOLE-
WHEAT PITA OR BREAD.

Salad
2 cups 1/2" cubes red boiling potatoes
2 cups 1/2" diagonal slices carrots
2 cups broccoli flowerets
2 cups 1/2" medium pieces cauliflower
2 cups 1/2" pieces green beans
2 cups frozen peas

Dressing
2 cups low-fat or nonfat cottage cheese
3 to 5 cloves garlic, sliced thin
1/4 cup powdered vegetable broth or onion powder
1/4 cup balsamic vinegar
2 tablespoons lemon juice
1 tablespoons low-sodium soy sauce
2 teaspoons dry mustard
1 teaspoon black pepper
1/4 cup minced fresh parsley

Fill a small pot half full of water and bring to a brisk boil. Add the
potatoes and simmer gently until soft, about 5 minutes. When done,
drain in a colander and cool.

Steaming time for vegetables depends on their consistency. Begin
with a large kettle, a little water, and the carrots. Steam for 3 minutes.
Add the broccoli and all of the other vegetables except the peas,
according to the following schedule: steaming time for broccoli and
cauliflower, 4 to 5 minutes, green beans, 2 to 3 minutes. Meanwhile,
cook the peas according to package directions. Drain all the vegetables and allow to cool.

In a food processor or blender, blend together all the ingredients for the dressing. Be sure to blend or process long enough so that the curds of the cottage cheese become velvety smooth.

When the vegetables are cool, place in a large bowl and gently toss with the dressing and parsley. The potatoes should mush slightly. Refrigerate for a few hours or overnight before serving.

Calories per serving: 150. Percent of calories from fat 5%, protein 31%, carbohydrates 64%, 2 mg cholesterol.

✳ *Cheese Salad*

Serves 4

LOW-FAT (2% MILKFAT) COTTAGE CHEESE IS AT ONCE LOW IN FAT, LOW IN CALORIES, AND EXTREMELY VERSATILE. THE NEW NONFAT VARIETY OF COTTAGE CHEESE MAY BE USED FOR AN EVEN LOWER-CALORIE, TOTALLY NONFAT VARIATION OF THIS DIET. HOWEVER, THE PRESENCE OF SOME PERCENTAGE OF FAT IN COTTAGE CHEESE IMPARTS A RICHER FLAVOR THAT YOU MIGHT PREFER. THE FEW ADDITIONAL CALORIES MIGHT BE WORTH IT TO YOU.

PRACTICALLY ANY COMBINATION OF VEGETABLES CAN BE SUBSTITUTED HERE. SIMPLY CHOP EVERYTHING QUITE FINE.

    4 large lettuce leaves
    2 cups low-fat or nonfat cottage cheese
    2 carrots, grated or diced
    1 fresh tomato, seeds removed, chopped
    1/2 cup grapes, sliced in half
    1/2 cup diced celery
    1/2 cup diced green bell pepper
    2 scallions, whites only, sliced thin
    2 tablespoons wheat bran
    2 tablespoons wheat germ
    Black pepper to taste

Set the lettuce leaves aside. Mix together all the remaining ingredients. Serve on the lettuce leaves.

Calories per serving: 150. Percent of calories from fat 13%, protein 44%, carbohydrates 42%, 5 mg cholesterol.

✳ *Hummus*

Serves 4, makes about 1 1/3 cups

COMMON NOW IN MOST METROPOLITAN AREAS, HUMMUS IS QUITE NUTRI-
TIOUS.   HOWEVER, THE TRADITIONAL RECIPE IS LOADED WITH OLIVE OIL.
WHILE OLIVE OIL IS THE HEALTHIEST OIL, IT IS STILL AS HIGH IN FAT AS OTHER
FATS AND OILS, AND YOU SHOULD LIMIT YOUR INTAKE.   OLIVE OIL IS SO FLA-
VORFUL THAT A LITTLE BIT GOES A VERY LONG WAY. WHEN YOU USE LESS, YOU
WILL FIND THAT YOUR DISHES ARE JUST AS FLAVORFUL AND MUCH LIGHTER.
YOUR TOTAL FAT CONTENT IS OF CHIEF CONCERN.   OUR HUMMUS IS A LOWER
FAT VERSION.
    HUMMUS MAKES A FINE DIP WITH BAKED TORTILLA CHIPS OR FRESH VEG-
ETABLES.   BAKE PITA POCKETS OR FLOUR TORTILLAS AND BREAK THEM INTO
CHIPS.   OR THIN THE HUMMUS DOWN WITH NONFAT YOGURT AND SERVE AS A
TOPPING FOR STEAMED VEGETABLES OR AS A SIDE DISH WITH PASTA.   TO EAT
AS A SANDWICH, PUT ONE SERVING OF HUMMUS INTO A PITA POCKET, OR ON TWO
SLICES OF WHOLE-GRAIN BREAD, WITH LETTUCE, TOMATO, AND ONION.

    1 1/3 cup drained canned garbanzo beans (chickpeas)
    1 clove garlic, or more to taste, pressed
    2 tablespoons lemon juice
    1 teaspoon low-sodium soy sauce
    1 tablespoon brewer's yeast
    Vegetable broth or water as needed
    1 carrot, grated
    4 scallions, whites only, minced
    1 tablespoon fresh parsley, minced
    Dash each of cayenne pepper and salt

In a food processor puree the beans, garlic, lemon juice, soy sauce and yeast, adding broth to make the consistency you desire. Transfer to a small bowl and stir in the carrot, scallions, parsley, cayenne, and salt.

Adjust to your taste by adding more garlic and/or cayenne.
Calories per serving: 130. Percent of calories from fat 9%, protein 22%, carbohydrates 69%, 0 mg cholesterol.

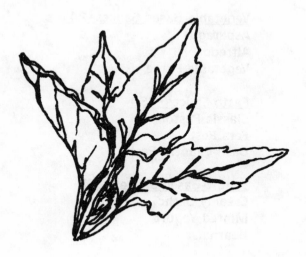

Sauces, Condiments and Relishes

VEGETABLE-BASED SAUCES

✳ *Asparagus Sauce*

Serves 5, makes about 1 2/3 cups

THIS SAUCE IS WONDERFUL ON FISH, CAULIFLOWER, OR PASTA. TO MAKE A SIMPLE PASTA TREAT, COOK WHOLE-WHEAT NOODLES, CHOP A FEW RIPE TOMATOES AND SOME FRESH BASIL, TOSS WITH THE PASTA, AND COVER WITH ASPARAGUS SAUCE.

2 bunches fresh asparagus, trimmed
2/3 cup nonfat (skim) milk
1/4 cup nonfat dry milk
2 tablespoons lemon juice
2 tablespoons salsa, bottled or homemade
1/4 cup chopped fresh cilantro
1 teaspoon dried marjoram

Steam the asparagus for 3 to 5 minutes depending on thickness. Put the asparagus and all the remaining ingredients except for the 2/3 cup nonfat milk into a food processor and puree. While pureeing, add the nonfat milk in a thin stream until you reach the consistency you want.

Calories per 1/3 cup serving: 47. Percent of calories from fat 4%, protein 35%, carbohydrates 61%, 9 mg cholesterol.

✳ *Alfredo Sauce*

Serves 12, makes about 4 cups

SERVE OVER PASTA WITH GREEN PEAS, CHOPPED RED PEPPERS, AND SCALLIONS.

1/2 large head cauliflower
1 cup low-fat or nonfat ricotta cheese
1 cup buttermilk
3 tablespoons grated Parmesan cheese
1 1/2 cups chicken or vegetable broth
1 clove garlic
1/2 teaspoon black pepper
Dash of paprika

Cut the cauliflower into bite-size pieces and steam for 5 minutes. In a food processor or a blender puree the cauliflower with all the other ingredients. Adjust seasonings to taste.

These quantities make a thick sauce. Use more broth for a lighter sauce, more buttermilk for a richer sauce.

Calories per 1/3 cup serving: 49. Percent of calories from fat 40%. protein 21%, carbohydrates 21%, 115 mg cholesterol.

✳ Vegetable Puree Sauce

Serves 4, makes about 2 cups

THIS SAUCE IS SO VERSATILE AND CREATIVE THAT YOU WILL WANT TO TRY IT ON EVERYTHING. WHETHER YOU ARE SERVING RICE AND VEGETABLES, BROILED FISH, LAMB CHOPS, OR MARINATED TOFU, SIMPLY MATCH UP AN APPROPRIATE VEGETABLE AND HERB INTO THE BASE OF THIS SAUCE.

THIS SAUCE CONTAINS APPROXIMATELY 50 CALORIES PER 1/2-CUP SERVING. IF YOU PREFER A RICHER SAUCE, ADD 1 TABLESPOON OF SOFTENED MARGARINE, WHICH WILL PUSH THE CALORIES PER SERVING UP TO ABOUT 70.

1 boiling potato, peeled
2 pounds vegetable of your choice
    (broccoli, carrots, asparagus, peas)
1/4 to 1/2 cup evaporated skim milk,
    depending on thickness desired
1/8 teaspoon seasonings of your choice (see note)
Dash of salt and pepper
1/2 clove garlic (optional)
1/8 teaspoon cayenne (optional)

Chop the potato and vegetable into large chunks. Combine in a large saucepan, cover with water, and boil for 12 to 15 minutes, or until quite soft. Drain well.

In a food processor, combine the potato and vegetable with the remaining ingredients and puree until smooth. Transfer to a blender if a smoother sauce is desired.

Just before serving, reheat the sauce over low heat and adjust the seasonings.

Note: Sample seasoning complements (use sparingly)— *asparagus*: marjoram, tarragon, lemon peel, paprika; *broccoli*: oregano, sweet basil, thyme, onion powder; *carrots*: marjoram, tarragon, dill, cumin, ginger, caraway; *peas*: tarragon, thyme, dill, marjoram, oregano.

Calories per 1/2 cup serving: 50. Percent of calories from fat 4%, protein 24%, carbohydrates 73%, 3 mg cholesterol.

PESTO SAUCES

✳ *Classic Pesto*

Serves 6, makes about 2 cups

PESTO IS AN ALL-TIME FAVORITE. WE'VE CASED LOS ANGELES TO FIND OUR FAVORITE PESTO, AND STILL RETURN TO THIS. MY TASTE BUDS FIND THAT THE FRAGRANCE OF FRESHLY MADE PESTO — THE BASIL, THE GARLIC — IS ENOUGH TO BUILD AN APPETITE. THE HEAVIER, OLIVE OIL-BASED PREPARATIONS NO LONGER HOLD ANY ALLURE FOR US. THIS RECIPE IS ADAPTABLE TO ALMOST ANY SPICY GREEN HERB SUCH AS CILANTRO, PARSLEY, SORREL, OR ARUGULA. VARY THE CHEESE TO COMPLEMENT THE HERB. OR OMIT THE CHEESE ENTIRELY AND ADD EXTRA SEEDS. TRADITIONAL PESTOS USE PINE NUTS, WHICH ARE EXTREMELY FATTY. TOASTED PUMPKIN SEEDS ARE RICHLY FLAVORED AND 50 PERCENT LIGHTER THAN PINE NUTS. EACH 1/3-CUP SERVING CONTAINS 100 CALORIES. EVEN BY OMITTING ALL OF THE OIL, PESTO STILL HAS A FAIRLY HIGH FAT CONTENT, 65 PERCENT. IF THIS IS A CONCERN, REDUCE THE CHEESE AND SEEDS BY HALF.

2 to 3 cloves garlic
2 cups packed fresh basil leaves
1/2 cup grated romano or Parmesan cheese
1/2 cup chicken broth
1/2 cup pumpkin seeds, toasted

Classic pesto should be coarse and crunchy. It is not really a cream sauce, so be careful not to overprocess. Of course, if you happen to prefer a creamy pesto, then process until smooth.

With the blade running in your food processor, add the garlic and run for 5 seconds. Turn the motor off and add all the basil. Run for 1 to 2 minutes, until chopped. Add all the remaining ingredients and process as briefly as possible, scraping the sides of the bowl often.

As this recipe has no oil at all, the liquids might rise to the top if the sauce sits for a while. If this occurs, simply stir.

Calories per one third cup serving: 100. Percent of calories from fat 65%, protein 30%, carbohydrates 9%, 6 mg cholesterol.

✳ *Feta Pesto*

Prepare as above, substituting feta cheese for the romano. Add 1/4 teaspoon black pepper.

See Classic Pesto (above) for nutritional profile.

✳ *Basil-Cilantro Pesto*

Prepare as for Basic Pesto, substituting 3/4 cup cilantro leaves for 3/4 cup of the basil leaves. Add a touch of salt. Toasted walnuts may be used instead of the pumpkin seeds.

See Classic Pesto (above) for nutritional profile.

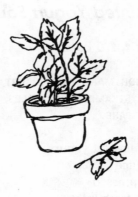

YOGURT-BASED SAUCES

✳ *Creamy Garlic Sauce*

Serves 5, makes about 1 2/3 cups

GREAT OVER BAKED POTATOES, STEAMED VEGETABLES, AND LAMB. THE GARLIC FLAVOR STRENGTHENS WITH TIME, SO ADJUST ACCORDINGLY THE NUMBER OF CLOVES YOU USE TO BOTH YOUR PALATE FOR GARLIC AND YOUR PROPOSED SERVING TIME.

1 cup plain nonfat or low-fat yogurt
1/2 cup soft tofu, plain kefir, or nonfat
    or low-fat sour cream
4 large cloves garlic, pressed
1/2 teaspoon prepared mustard

Mix all the ingredients thoroughly together in a blender or with a whisk. Heat in a small saucepan over low heat for 5 minutes. Serve immediately.

Calories per 1/3 cup serving: 52. Percent of calories from fat 30%, protein 34%, carbohydrates 35%, 15 mg cholesterol.

✳ *Minted Yogurt Sauce*

Serves 4, makes about 1 1/3 cups

FRESH MINT AND LEMON MAKE THIS YOGURT SAUCE A REALLY SUPERB ACCOMPANIMENT FOR FISH, STEAMED VEGETABLES, GRAIN DISHES AND EVEN PASTA. IT IS SIMPLE TO PREPARE.

1 cup plain nonfat or low-fat yogurt
1 tablespoon lemon juice
2 large cloves garlic, pressed
3 tablespoons minced fresh mint

Dash of white pepper
Curry powder to taste

Mix all the ingredients together with a fork and serve either cold or
gently heated.

Calories per 1/3 cup serving: 43. Percent of calories from fat 20%,
protein 31%, carbohydrates 48%, 15 mg cholesterol.

gently heated.

Calories per 1/3 cup serving: 43. Percent of calories from fat 20%,
protein 31%, carbohydrates 48%, 15 mg cholesterol.

✳ *Bearnaise Sauce*

Serves 5, makes about 1 2/3 cups

WITH ONLY A QUARTER THE CALORIES OF ITS ORIGINAL BUTTER-BASED
COUSIN, YOU CAN SERVE THIS SAUCE LIBERALLY OVER MEAT OR FISH.

1/2 cup dry white wine
2 tablespoons tarragon vinegar
3 scallions, whites only, minced
1 tablespoon chopped fresh tarragon
    or 2 teaspoons dried
1 tablespoon chopped fresh marjoram
    or 2 teaspoons dried
1/4 teaspoon black pepper
1/2 teaspoon prepared horseradish
    or 1 teaspoon prepared mustard
2/3 cup plain low-fat or nonfat yogurt
2 tablespoons minced fresh parsley
2 tablespoons fresh herbs
    (dill for fish; rosemary or oregano for meat)

In a small saucepan combine the wine, vinegar, scallions, tarragon, marjoram, and pepper. Simmer for 10 minutes, lower the heat, then strain. To the juices add the horseradish. Cool for 5 minutes, then mix in the yogurt, parsley, and herbs to taste. May be gently heated or served cool.

Calories per 1/3 cup serving: 34. Percent of calories from fat 20%, protein 31%, carbohydrates 48%, 15 mg cholesterol.

TOFU-BASED SAUCES

TOFU HAS A VERY CREAMY TEXTURE AND ASSUMES FLAVORS EASILY. THIS CHARACTERISTIC MAKES IT A GOOD BASE FOR MANY THINGS, FROM TOPPINGS FOR MOUSSAKA AND QUICHES, TO SALAD DRESSINGS AND SAUCES. THE SOFT VARIETY OF TOFU WHIPS UP WELL.

☀ Sesame Sauce

Serves 4, makes about 1 1/2 cups

   1/4 cup sesame tahini
   1/4 cup water
   2 cloves garlic, peeled
   2 tablespoon rice vinegar
   1 teaspoon low-sodium soy sauce
   1 teaspoon lemon juice
   Black pepper to taste
   8 ounces soft tofu, drained

Blend the first 7 ingredients in a food processor or blender until smooth. Add the tofu. Blend for 30 seconds.

Calories per 1/3 cup serving: 90. Percent of calories from fat 66%, protein 18%, carbohydrates 16%, 0 mg cholesterol.

✳ *Cream Sauce*

Serves 5, makes about 1 2/3 cups

HERBS OF YOUR CHOICE MAY BE ADDED.

8 ounces soft tofu
1/2 cup plain nonfat or low-fat yogurt
1 tablespoon sesame tahini
1 tablespoon miso or 1 clove garlic, peeled
1 tablespoon lemon juice

Blend all ingredients together in a blender.

Calories per 1/3 cup serving: 55. Percent of calories from fat 54%, protein 30%, carbohydrates 16%, 0 mg cholesterol.

✳ *Tartare Sauce*

Serves 5, makes about 1 2/3 cups

8 ounces soft tofu
2 tablespoons red wine vinegar
1 tablespoon olive oil
1 teaspoon honey
2 tablespoon sweet pickle relish
1/2 teaspoon prepared mustard
1/4 cup minced onion

Blend the tofu, vinegar, oil, and honey in a food processor or blender until smooth. Gently but thoroughly stir the relish, mustard, and onion into the tofu mixture.

Calories per 1/4 cup serving: 75. Percent of calories from fat 65%, protein 9%, carbohydrates 26%, 0 mg cholesterol.

GRAVY

Serves 8, makes about 2 cups

WHEN YOU HAVE SEVERAL COOKS IN THE FAMILY, HOLIDAYS CAN BECOME REAL FEAST DAYS! FOR THANKSGIVING WE HAD FOUR DIFFERENT KINDS OF STUFFING, A TURKEY, A VEGETARIAN LENTIL LOAF, MASHED POTATOES, PLENTY OF VEGETABLES, AND TWO KINDS OF GRAVY. EVERYONE TRIED THE FOLLOWING BREWER'S YEAST-BASED GRAVY ALONG WITH THE STANDARD, AND EVERYONE TOOK SECONDS OF BOTH. THIS GRAVY WHIPS UP IN MINUTES AND CAN BE SERVED WITH BISCUITS, BEEF, TOFU, AND BAKED POTATO.

THIS WILL KEEP WELL IN THE REFRIGERATOR FOR A WEEK.

1/4 cup whole-wheat flour
2 tablespoons olive oil
1 1/3 cups vegetable broth
2 tablespoons brewer's yeast
1/4 teaspoon dried oregano
1/4 teaspoon dried thyme or, for turkey, sage
1/2 teaspoon soy or Worcestershire sauce
Juice of 1/2 lemon
2 teaspoons arrowroot mixed
    with 2 teaspoons water, as needed

In a medium-size saucepan heat the flour for 3 minutes over low heat, or until it smells toasted. Slowly stir in the olive oil, coating the flour completely. Gradually dribble in the vegetable broth, a quarter cup at a time, stirring constantly with a fork or whisk to avoid lumps. When all of the broth has been added, stir in the yeast along with the herbs, soy sauce, and lemon juice.

If the sauce is too thick, add more vegetable broth. If it is too thin, add the arrowroot mixture to the gravy. Repeat as necessary to reach the thickness you like.

Calories per 1/4 cup serving: 30. Percent of calories from fat 35%, protein 21%, carbohydrates 15%, 0 mg cholesterol.

Vegetables

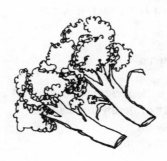

❊ Dilled Broccoli and Carrots

Serves 4

Olive oil cooking spray
2 tablespoons dry white wine
3 carrots, cut in 1/2" rounds
1 cup broccoli, flowerets only
2 teaspoons fresh minced dill or 1/2 teaspoon dried

Spray a skillet with olive oil.

Add the wine and heat over medium heat. Add the carrots and cook, covered, for 5 minutes.

Add the broccoli and dill and simmer another 5 minutes or until the vegetables are tender yet crisp.

Calories per serving: 60. Percentage of calories from fat 6%, protein 29%, carbohydrates 65%, 0 mg cholesterol.

❊ Broccoli Stems with Peas

Serves 4

BROCCOLI STEMS ARE LOADED WITH VITAMIN C. THEY MAKE AN EXCEL-LENT ADDITION TO ANY STEW OR CASSEROLE, AND CAN BE SERVED INDEPEN-DENTLY, AS IN THE FOLLOWING RECIPE.

SLICE AND DISCARD THE THICK OUTER SKIN AND YOU WILL SERVE, ONCE COOKED, A DELICACY SIMILIAR TO ARTICHOKE HEARTS.

Olive oil cooking spray
2 cups peeled broccoli stems
1/2 cup orange juice
2 cups fresh green peas or 1 package (10 ounces) frozen
5 scallions, including part of green tops, sliced
1/2 teaspoon dried marjoram
2 teaspoons fresh parsley, chopped

Heat a nonstick skillet sprayed with olive oil over medium heat.
Add the broccoli and half of the orange juice. Cover and
simmer for 5 minutes. Add the peas, scallions, remaining orange juice, and the marjoram, and cook, uncovered,
for an additional 3 to 5 minutes.
Serve topped with parsley.

Calories per serving: 100. Percentage of calories from fat 5%, protein 30%, carbohydrates 65%, 0 mg cholesterol.

✳ *Brussels Sprouts in Orange Sauce*

Serves 4

1 pound brussels sprouts
1 cup water
1/2 teaspoon marjoram
1 1/2 teaspoon cornstarch or arrowroot
1/4 cup orange juice
1 orange, peeled, seeded, and separated into sections
1/4 cup fresh cilantro, chopped

Cut a little cross into the base of each sprout. Combine
the sprouts, water, and the marjoram in a saucepan and cook,
covered, for 15 to 20 minutes, until the sprouts are tender. Drain and
set aside.
In a small saucepan, combine the cornstarch and orange juice. Heat
over low heat stirring constantly, until thickened. Add the orange sections and cook until bubbly. Pour over the drained sprouts and serve
garnished with cilantro.

Calories per serving: 80. Percentage of calories from fat 5%, protein
30%, carbohydrates 65%, 0 mg cholesterol.

☀ Minted Beets and Apples

Serves 4

THIS DISH IS GOOD SERVED COLD (MARINATED FOR 30 MINUTES) OR
WARM, JUST AFTER THE BEETS HAVE COOKED.

11/2 cups beets, peeled and quartered
1 large green apple, cored and diced fine
1/3 cup plain low-fat or nonfat yogurt
1 tablespoon minced fresh mint

In a small saucepan, steam the beets for 7 minutes or until tender.
Mix with the remaining ingredients and serve.

Calories per serving: 60. Percentage of calories from fat 9%, protein
15%, carbohydrates 76%, 2 mg cholesterol.

☀ Stir-Fried Cabbage with Leeks and Mushrooms

Serves 4

Olive oil cooking spray
2 tablespoons vegetable broth
1 teaspoon onion powder
2 large leeks, green tops trimmed off
    and well washed
1 cup fresh mushrooms, sliced thin
1/2 head green cabbage, sliced thin
1 teaspoon apple cider vinegar
1 teaspoon caraway seeds

Spray a large nonstick skillet with olive oil and heat over low heat.
Add the 2 tablespoons broth, the onion powder, leeks and mushrooms.
Cover, and simmer for 3 minutes. Remove the cover, and continue to
cook, stirring frequently, until the leeks are soft. Remove the leeks and

mushrooms from the skillet with a slotted spoon and set aside.

Add the remaining broth along with the cabbage to the skillet.

Cook, covered, over low heat for 5 to 7 minutes. Add the vinegar. Remove the cover and continue to cook until tender.

Return the leeks and mushrooms to the skilled along with the caraway seeds. Heat gently.

Calories per serving: 34. Percentage of calories from fat 6%, protein 20%, carbohydrates 73%, 0 mg cholesterol.

✳ *Baked Cabbage*

Serves 4

A CRUCIFEROUS VEGETABLE, CABBAGE IS ONE OF THE MORE NUTRITIOUS. CRUCIFEROUS VEGETABLES ARE IMMUNE SYSTEM STIMULATORS, AND ARE ALSO HIGH IN FIBER.

    4 1/2 cups vegetable broth or water
    1 cup barley
    Olive oil cooking spray
    4 cups (1 medium head) shredded green cabbage
    1/4 cup wheat germ
    1/2 teaspoon poppy seeds
    Seasonings of your choice—
        dill, marjoram, black pepper, etc.(optional)
    Dash of paprika

In a medium-size pot, bring 4 cups of the broth to a boil. Add the barley, cover the pot, and reduce the heat. Simmer for 25 minutes, or until done.

Spray a large flameproof casserole with olive oil. Over medium heat, add the remaining 1/2 cup broth and the cabbage. Sauté for 15 minutes, stirring frequently.

Add the barley, wheat germ, poppy seeds, and optional seasonings, then sprinkle paprika over the top.

Bake for 10 to 15 minutes, taste testing after 10 minutes. If the casserole bakes too long, the barley will dry out, so beware! Serve hot.

Calories per serving: 133. Percentage of calories from fat 7%, protein 14%, carbohydrates 79%, 0 mg cholesterol.

✳ *Corn Cakes*

Serves 4

> 11/2 cup fresh or frozen corn kernels,
>   thawed if frozen
> 4 egg whites
> 1 teaspoon wheat germ
> 2 tablespoons chopped scallions or
>   2 tablespoons fresh parsley, chopped
> 1/2 teaspoon ground cumin
> Canola oil cooking spray

Heat the oven to 350°F.

In a small food processor, cream half of the corn.

Whip the egg whites in a large bowl with a whisk until frothy. Fold in the creamed corn, whole kernel corn, wheat germ, scallions or parsley, and cumin.

Spray an 8-inch cast iron skillet with canola oil. Over a low heat pour in the corn mixture and cook until the edges set, then place in the oven for 15 minutes, or until set.

Cut into wedges to serve.

Calories per wedge: 90. Percentage of calories from fat 8%, protein 19%, carbohydrates 73%, 0 mg cholesterol.

✳ *Curried Vegetables*

Serves 4

SERVE THIS WITH RICE OR MILLET.

Olive oil cooking spray
1 small onion, sliced thin
2 tablespoons fresh ginger, peeled and minced
2 cloves garlic, peeled
1 small jalapeño chili, seeded and minced
1/2 teaspoon ground cardamom
1/2 cup vegetable broth or water
1/4 teaspoon ground turmeric
1 fresh tomato, chopped
2 medium-size potatoes, peeled
      and cut into 1/2" cubes
2 cups cauliflower flowerets
5 carrots, sliced into 1/2" rounds
2 cups fresh or frozen peas
1/2 cup low-fat or nonfat yogurt

Spray a large kettle with olive oil and sauté the onion slices over medium-high heat until golden. Meanwhile, puree the ginger, garlic, and chili in a food processor. Add to the onion along with the turmeric and stir-fry for a few minutes. Stir in the cardomom, broth, and all the vegetables except the peas.

Lower the heat to medium, cover, and cook for 20 minutes. Add the peas and continue to cook, uncovered, until all the liquid has evaporated. Gently stir in the yogurt. Heat through and serve.

Calories per serving: 115. Percentage of calories from fat 4%, protein 18%, carbohydrates 79%, 1 mg cholesterol.

✳ Szechwanese Eggplant

Serves 4

SERVE HOT, OVER NOODLES OR RICE

2 medium-size eggplants
1/2 cup chicken broth
2 teaspoons dry red wine
2 teaspoons low-sodium soy sauce
2 teaspoons rice vinegar
1/2 teaspoon sesame oil
1/4 teaspoon Tabasco, or to taste (optional)
1 teaspoon cornstarch mixed with 2 tablespoons water
1 tablespoon fresh ginger, peeled and minced
1 tablespoon minced garlic
2 tablespoons thinly sliced scallions, whites only

Preheat the oven to 350°F.

Cut the eggplant into strips 1/4" thick, and 2 to 3 inches long. Soak in cold water for 10 minutes while you prepare the sauce. For the sauce, mix the broth, wine, soy sauce, vinegar, 1/2 teaspoon of the sesame oil, and Tabasco, and set within easy reach of the stove.

Drain the eggplant, pat dry and place on a nonstick cookie sheet. Bake for 15 minutes, or until tender. Cool and cut into bite-size pieces.

Coat a large nonstick skillet lightly with the remaining 1/2 teaspoon sesame oil. Heat until a drop of water bounces across the pan, but avoid a smoking pan. Add the ginger, garlic, and scallions, and stir-fry quickly in the hot oil, 15 seconds. Reduce the heat to medium low. Stir in the eggplant and pour in the prepared sauce. Stir and cook for 5 minutes. Drizzle in the cornstarch mixture, stirring constantly. Increase the heat to medium and cook until the sauce thickens. Serve immediately.

Calories per serving: 40. Percentage of calories from fat 37%, protein 10%, carbohydrates 52%, 0 mg cholesterol.

✳ Potatoes

SINCE U.S.CITIZENS CONSUME ABOUT 130 POUNDS OF POTATOES PER PER-
SON EVERY YEAR, AND BECAUSE POTATOES ARE EXTREMELY NUTRITIOUS IN
THEIR NATURAL STATE, HERE ARE SEVERAL WAYS OF PREPARING THEM THAT DO
NOT ADD MANY CALORIES.

Baked potato: Bake in the oven for 45 minutes, or in the
microwave for 5 minutes. Dress with chopped scallions plus low-fat
yogurt or with low-fat cottage cheese mixed with diced bell peppers
and sliced onions.

Simple stuffed potato: Cut a large baked potato in half (either
lengthwise or crosswise), scoop out the pulp and mash with 1/3 cup of
low-fat cottage cheese and two tablespoons each chopped scallions
and parsley. Fill the potato shells with this mixture and sprinkle with 1
to 2 teaspoons of grated Parmesan cheese. Reheat briefly in the
microwave.

Scalloped potatoes: Slice the raw potato, leaving on the peel, into
1/4" slices. Layer alternately with sliced onion in a casserole, sprinkling
each layer with pepper and a little flour. Dot with a very small amount
of margarine and pour 1 cup of nonfat or low-fat milk over the slices.
Microwave on high for 7 to 8 minutes.

Mashed potatoes: Add warm buttermilk (instead of whole milk
and butter) to boiled potatoes and mash. The mashed potatoes will
have a slightly buttery taste but without the fat.

❈ Sweet Potato Salad

Serves 8

YOU MAY SUBSTITUTE BAKING POTATOES FOR HALF THE SWEET POTATOES. WHILE BROILING, COVER THE BAKING POTATOES WITH PLENTY OF MINCED GARLIC.

THIS DISH CAN BE SERVED HOT OR COLD AND WILL KEEP IN THE REFRIGERATOR FOR A WEEK. THE SWEET POTATOES TEND TO BE MOISTER AND HENCE MAKE A BETTER SALAD, WHILE THE COMBINATION OF THE TWO IS GREAT FOR A HOT DISH.

4 large sweet potatoes or 2 large sweet
    and 2 large russet potatoes, scrubbed
Canola oil cooking spray
Dash of cayenne pepper or ground cinnamon
1/4 cup raspberry vinegar
    or any slightly fruity vinegar
1/4 cup balsamic vinegar
2 tablespoons low-sodium soy sauce
1/4 cup vegetable broth or water
8 scallions, whites only, sliced thin
1/2 teaspoon black pepper
2 red bell peppers, seeded and chopped fine

Preheat the broiler.

Fill a large stockpot one fourth full of water and bring to a boil. Slice the potatoes into 1/2" rounds. Add to the pot and parboil for 6 to 8 minutes, until the potatoes can barely be pierced with a fork. Remove the pot from the flame and strain out the cooking liquids (which make a wonderful broth for soup).

Lay each potato slice on a rack in a broiler pan and spray lightly with canola oil. Sprinkle sweet potatoes with cayenne or cinnamon and broil for 5 minutes, until blackened but not dehydrated. Watch closely, as you may lose the entire dish if the potatoes are broiled for too long. Remove from the broiler and turn the potatoes over. If using russets, cover with 3 cloves fresh minced garlic, then return all potatoes to broiler for 3 or 4 minutes. Remove from the heat and allow to cool.

In a large bowl mix the vinegars, soy sauce, broth, scallions, and black pepper.

Cut the potatoes into 1/2" cubes and add to the dressing along with the bell peppers. Toss gently, but thoroughly. If you are serving the salad cold, cover the bowl with plastic wrap and marinate for at least 1 hour.

Calories per serving: 112. Percentage of calories from fat 3%, protein 7%, carbohydrates 90%, 0 mg cholesterol.

✳ Sweet Potatoes and Chestnuts

Serves 8

2 pounds yams or sweet potatoes
1/2 lb frozen or bottled whole chestnuts
2 fresh, ripe pears
1/4 cup water
1/4 cup maple syrup
Juice of 1 orange

Preheat oven to 350°F.

Bake the potatoes for 45 minutes. Cool for 15 minutes, then peel. Halve lengthwise, then slice into 1/2" rounds.

While the potatoes are baking, peel the pears, core and chop. Place in a small saucepan with the water, maple syrup, and orange juice. Heat over medium heat until hot, then reduce the heat and simmer for 30 minutes.

In a large baking dish combine the potatoes, pears, and whole chestnuts and gently mix.

Bake for 15 to 20 minutes, or until bubbly.

Calories per serving: 158. Percentage of calories from fat 4%, protein 5%, carbohydrates 91%, 0 mg cholesterol.

CHARD, KALE, SPINACH, AND BEET, MUSTARD, AND TURNIP GREENS ARE RICH IN CALCIUM, VITAMIN A AND IRON. WHEN BUYING GREENS, LOOK FOR LEAVES THAT ARE FREE FROM BLEMISHES AND HAVE A RICH GREEN COLOR.

IF YOU ARE NEW TO GREENS TRY EACH SEPARATELY. WITH UNIQUE FLAVORS RANGING FROM MUSTARD GREENS' SPICY BITE TO TURNIP GREENS' RICH, AND MILDLY SALTY FLAVOR TO THE ROBUSTNESS OF KALE, GREENS ARE A VARIED LOT. SIMPLY STEAM THEM, AND SPRINKLE ON A LITTLE BALSAMIC OR RASPBERRY VINEGAR. OR TRY THE RECIPES BELOW.

✳ *Sherried Swiss Chard*

Serves 4

   1 1/2 pounds Swiss chard, rinsed and drained
      Olive oil cooking spray
   1 clove garlic, minced
   1/4 cup dry sherry
   1 teaspoon grated Parmesan cheese

Cut the white stalks from the chard leaves, chop, and set aside. Chop the leaves.

Begin steaming the stalks for 5 minutes, then add the leaves and continue steaming another 10 minutes.

Drain the chard. Spray a large nonstick skillet with olive oil. Add the garlic and dry-fry for 1 minute. Add the sherry and chard and stir thoroughly. Simmer for 5 minutes.

Transfer to a serving dish, add the cheese, and toss gently.

Calories per serving: 56. Percentage of calories from fat 25%, protein 30%, carbohydrates 45%, 5 mg cholesterol.

✳ Shiitake Mushrooms and Greens

Serves 4

1 1/2 pounds beet, turnip, or mustard greens
4 large fresh shiitake mushrooms or
    6 dried, soaked for 20 minutes and drained
Olive oil cooking spray
1 clove garlic, pressed
1/2 small red onion, sliced thin
Dash of low-sodium soy sauce

Wash, rinse, and chop the greens. Slice the mushrooms into long thin slices.

Spray a large nonstick skillet with olive oil. Over low heat, cook the garlic, onion, and mushrooms, adding drizzles of water as needed. Sprinkle with soy sauce and simmer for 5 minutes.

Add the greens. Cover and simmer for 10 minutes, or until done

Calories per serving: 77. Percentage of calories from fat 6%, protein 23%, carbohydrates 70%, 0 mg cholesterol.

✳ Greens Soup

Serves 4

4 cups chicken or vegetable broth
3 thin slices fresh ginger
1/2 teaspoon low-sodium soy sauce
1/2 teaspoon honey
1 large bunch mustard greens or spinach,
    well washed and coarsely chopped

Combine broth, ginger, soy sauce, and honey in a large saucepan and simmer for 15 minutes.

Add the greens to the broth and bring the soup to a full boil.

Reduce the heat, cover, and simmer 5 to 7 minutes, depending on which greens you selected. Remove the ginger slices before serving.

Calories per serving: 47, Percentage of calories from fat 6%, protein 25%, carbohydrates 70%, 0 mg cholesterol.

✳ *Creamed Greens Soup*

Prepare Greens Soup (above). After removing the ginger slices, puree the cooked soup in a food processor or blender and add to it, stirring constantly, 1/2 cup instant powdered nonfat milk.

Calories per serving: 100. Percentage of calories from fat 7%, protein 35%, carbohydrates 42%, 0 mg cholesterol.

✳ *Spinach and Roasted Garlic*

Serves 4

YOU MAY HAVE TASTED IN AN ITALIAN RESTAURANT ESCAROLE WITH GAR-
LIC AND OIL WHICH USES THE SAME AMOUNT OF GARLIC AS WE DO HERE.
GARLIC MELLOWS AS IT COOKS. FRESH SPINACH REALLY MAKES THE DIFFER-
ENCE WITH THIS RECIPE. AND DON'T BE FRIGHTENED BY ALL THE GARLIC! ITS
PUNGENCY MELLOWS WITH COOKING. TO SAVE TIME, YOU MIGHT BUY PREM-
INCED GARLIC.

   Olive oil cooking spray
   2 large bunches fresh spinach, washed,
      left undrained, torn to bite-size
   10 large cloves garlic, minced
   1 teaspoon low-sodium soy sauce
   1/4 teaspoon dried marjoram
   1/4 teaspoon grated lemon peel

Spray a large nonstick skillet with olive oil and heat over medium heat. Add the spinach with the water clinging to the leaves and garlic and cook, covered, over a low flame for 5 minutes. Remove the cover and add the soy sauce and other seasonings. Stir and simmer until the liquid is absorbed, another 3 minutes. The spinach should still be bright in color.

Calories per serving: 16. Percentage of calories from fat 8%, protein 38%, carbohydrates 54%, 0 mg cholesterol.

✳ *Caramelized Butternut Squash*

Serves 4

1 medium-size butternut
   or kabochi squash
Canola oil cooking spray
2 cloves garlic, pressed
1 onion, sliced thin, in rings
1 tablespoon mirin (Japanese rice wine)
   or dry sherry
1 teaspoon raspberry vinegar
1/2 teaspoon walnut oil
Dash of soy sauce
1/2 teaspoon fresh rosemary,
   or1 teaspoon dried

Preheat the oven to 350°F.

Bake the squash for 30 minutes to soften. Peel, seed, and slice into large, chunky pieces.

Spray a nonstick skillet with canola oil and caramelize the garlic and onion, adding the mirin, vinegar, walnut oil, soy sauce and rosemary. Add a little water if the dry-fry dries out.

Add the squash to the skillet and simmer for 20 minutes.

Stir infrequently, adding extra water only if the squash dries out, forming a glaze over it.

Calories per serving: 114. Percentage of calories from fat 20%, protein 8%, carbohydrates 71%, 0 mg cholesterol.

✳ Mixed Summer Squash

Serves 4

1/4 cup water
2 zucchini, sliced into 1/2" rounds
2 yellow crookneck squash, halved and
    sliced into 1/2" pieces
1 clove garlic, pressed
1 tablespoon lemon juice
Dash each of pepper and dried dill

Put the 1/4 cup water in a small saucepan, add the two squashes and the garlic, and simmer for 3 minutes, until tender yet crisp. Drain off any unabsorbed liquids and add the remaining ingredients. Stir well and reheat. Serve immediately.

Calories per serving: 26. Percentage of calories from fat 4%, protein 19%, carbohydrates 76%, 0 mg cholesterol.

✳ Herbed Spaghetti Squash

Serves 4

THIS VEGETABLE IMPERSONATES SPAGHETTI SO WELL THAT WE FREQUENT-LY MIX IT WITH SPAGHETTI WHEN WE WANT A LIGHTER PASTA. THE STRANDS OF YELLOW-ORANGE CRUNCHY VEGETABLE SLIP OUT OF THE SHELL EASILY ONLY AFTER BAKING FOR 40 TO 50 MINUTES. CHILDREN LOVE THIS ONE.

1 large spaghetti squash (about 3 pounds)
1 cup low-fat or nonfat cottage cheese
1 tablespoon fresh parsley, minced
1/2 teaspoon dried oregano
1/4 teaspoon dried thyme
Dash of black pepper

Preheat the oven to 350°F.

Place the squash in a large baking pan and bake for 20 minutes. Remove, cut in half, discard the seeds, and return to the pan along with the 1/4 cup of the water. Continue baking for another 20 to 30 minutes, or until the spaghetti-like strands lift out of the shell easily.

Place the cottage cheese in a blender or food processor and blend or process until velvety smooth.

Stir all the remaining ingredients into the cheese, then add to the squash and heat, stirring constantly, over a low flame until hot.

Calories per serving: 146. Percentage of calories from fat 7%, protein 25%, carbohydrates 67%, 3 mg cholesterol.

✳ *Stuffed Tomatoes*

Serves 4

4 medium-size fresh tomatoes
Olive oil cooking spray
1/4 green bell pepper, seeded and diced
1/2 red onion, minced
1/4 cup whole-wheat bread crumbs
2 tablespoons wheat germ
2 tablespoons chopped black olives
2 tablespoons parsley
1 egg white
Dash each of salt and black pepper

Preheat the oven to 350°F.

Core each tomato, and carefully hollow it out so that you have an intact tomato shell. Retain the pulp. Turn each shell upside down on paper towels to drain. Separate the wet seeds from the pulp, discard the seeds and chop the pulp.

Spray a small nonstick skillet with olive oil. Dry-fry the green pepper and onion, adding water if needed. Add the tomato pulp, bread crumbs, and wheat germ and stir well.

Remove from the heat, and mix in the olives, parsley, and egg-white, salt and pepper.

Stuff each tomato cup, and bake for 30 minutes.

Calories per serving: 52. Percentage of calories from fat 18%, protein 14%, carbohydrates 67%, 0 mg cholesterol.

✳ Spiced Tomatoes

Serves 4

THIS SIDE DISH ADDS DIMENSION TO ANY GRAIN-CENTERED MEAL. I HAVE SERVED IT ALONGSIDE RICE WITH FISH, CHICKEN, AND VEGETARIAN COMBINATIONS. THE EXOTIC BLACK MUSTARD SEEDS TRANSFORM THE SIMPLE TOMATOES INTO A RICH SAUCE THAT IS LUSCIOUS WHEN SPOONED OVER GRAINS.

Olive oil cooking spray
1 clove garlic
1/4 onion, minced
1/2 teaspoon cumin seeds
1 teaspoon whole black mustard seeds
1 dried red pepper, whole
4 large fresh ripe tomatoes, peeled
1 tsp peeled ginger, minced
Dash of black pepper
1 tablespoon whole-wheat flour
    mixed with 2 tablespoons water

Spray a large nonstick skillet with olive oil and place over medium heat. Add the garlic and onion and sauté. Remove with a slotted spoon. Add the cumin and black mustard seeds to the skillet. In a few seconds, when the seeds begin to pop, add the red pepper and tomatoes. Cover and lower heat to low. Add the ginger and black pepper, cover, and simmer for 8 minutes. Whisk in the flour/water mixture and keep whisking until it has thoroughly blended into the tomatoes.

Serve hot.

Calories per serving: 37. Percentage of calories from fat 6%, protein 16%, carbohydrates 78%, 0 mg cholesterol.

✳ Broiled Vegetables

Serves 4

OFTEN THE SIMPLEST TECHNIQUES ARE THE BEST. IN THIS CASE, BROILED VEGETABLES ARE QUICK AND EASY TO PREPARE, AND CAN ACCOMPANY MOST ANY MAIN DISH ELEGANTLY.   DIFFERENT VEGETABLES NEED TO BE DIFFERENTLY BROILED, AND ALL VEGETABLES, WHEN PROPERLY CUT, SPRAYED OR BRUSHED WITH CANOLA OIL, AND CAREFULLY WATCHED IN THE OVEN, WILL REMAIN MOIST. MUSHROOMS, EGGPLANT, ONIONS, RED PEPPERS, TOMATOES AND ZUCCHINI ARE SUCCULANT AND MOIST IN THEMSELVES.   ROOT VEGIES, LIKE SWEET POTATOES, BEETS, AND TURNIPS, NEED TO BE PARBOILED PRIOR TO BROILING.   THE SEASONING CAN VARY FROM VEGETABLE TO VEGETABLE.   TRY SEASONING THE ONIONS WITH RED PEPPER, THE EGGPLANT WITH OREGANO, AND THE MUSHROOMS WITH DILL OR TARRAGON.

1 medium eggplant, sliced into 1/2" rounds
Salt
Canola oil cooking spray
1 red bell pepper, halved, and seeded
1 large red onion,
       sliced into 1/4"rounds
1 large zucchini,
       sliced into 1/2" rounds
12 to 15 medium-size fresh mushrooms, stemmed
Seasonings of your choice:
       cayenne pepper, oregano, sweet basil, coriander,
       celery salt, onion, garlic powder
Balsamic or tarragon vinegar
8 cherry tomatoes
Low-sodium soy sauce
Water

Preheat the broiler.

Sprinkle each eggplant slice with salt and set aside in a bowl for 10 minutes. This leaches out the bitter juices.

Spray the rack in a broiler pan with canola oil. Arrange all of the bell pepper and as many of the onion slices and zucchini as will fit in the pan. Lightly spray or brush the vegetables with canola oil; dribble on a little soy sauce. Sprinkle the seasoning of your choice over the vegetables.

Place the pan under the broiler for 4 minutes, brushing the vegetables halfway through with balsamic vinegar. Check for doneness. The best way I've found is the old-fashioned taste test.

When the bell pepper halves turn black, remove them from the broiler and place in a plastic bag. Blow some air into the bag to puff it up, and set aside for 6 or 7 minutes. Then peel the blackened skin off the peppers.

When the first batch of vegetables is broiled to your liking (6 minutes for crisp vegetables), repeat the process with the remaining vegetables — the eggplant, mushrooms and cherry tomatoes — in a second patch. If you have a very large oven, all of the vegetables can be broiled at once. Just be sure that they are not so crowded that they overlap, as you want each vegetable to be exposed to the broiler.

As you remove the cooked vegetables from the broiler, brush again with a diluted mixture of soy sauce, water, and balsamic vinegar and keep warm on a warm, covered plate.

When all of the vegetables are cooked, serve immediately with rice and Sesame Sauce.

Calories per serving: 64. Percentage of calories from fat 7%, protein 18%, carbohydrates 76%, 0 mg cholesterol.

Desserts

❊ Chocolate Layer Cake

Serves 12

AND THESE ARE NOT EENTSY-BEENTSY PIECES EITHER! WE RECOMMEND THE CAKE WITH ANY VARIETY OF ALL-FRUIT JAM OR PRESERVES SPREAD BETWEEN THE LAYERS. YOU COULD ALSO SPOON YOUR FAVORITE LIQUEUR OVER THE TOP OR DUST IT LIGHTLY WITH A SIFTING OF POWDERED SUGAR.

Canola oil cooking spray
1 1/2 cups oat flour
1/4 cup nonfat dry milk
1/4 cup unsweetened cocoa powder
1/2 teaspoon baking soda
1/4 cup cornstarch
Dash of salt
1/4 cup ground almonds
4 egg whites
3/4 cup honey
1 teaspoon vanilla
1 cup water
1/3 cup any all-fruit
     (unsweetened) preserves or jam

Preheat oven to 350°F. Spray two 9-inch cake pans with canola oil.

Sift the dry ingredients into a medium bowl and mix in the ground almonds.

In a large bowl combine the egg whites, honey and vanilla. Beat well. Stir in the flour mixture alternately with the water, beginning and ending with water.

Pour the batter into the prepared cake pans. Bake for 30 minutes, or until a toothpick inserted in the center comes out clean. Cool in the pan for 5 minutes, then invert onto a wire cooling rack.

When totally cooled, spread the bottom layer with the preserves or jam. Stack the second layer on top.

Calories per serving: 157. Percent of calories from fat 19%, protein 11%, carbohydrates 70%, 0 mg cholesterol.

✳ *Spiced Honey Cake*

Proceed as in the recipe for Chocolate Layer Cake (above), with the following modifications: Substitute 1 cup whole-wheat flour for 1 cup of the oat flour and omit the cocoa powder. Use 1/4 cup toasted minced walnuts instead of the almonds. Minced nuts added to the batter will give a crunchier texture. Add 1/2 teaspoon ground cinnamon and 1/4 teaspoon ground allspice.

This cake is delicious served with sliced kiwis in between the two layers and fresh strawberries on top or with Apple Butter.

Calories per serving (for cake alone): 118. Percent of calories from fat 13%, protein 12%, carbohydrates 75%, 5 mg cholesterol.

✳ Maple Angel Food Cake

Serves 12

THIS CAKE, DUSTED WITH A SIFTING OF POWDERED SUGAR, IS DECORA-
TIVELY BEAUTIFUL AT HOLIDAY TIMES. SERVED PLAIN, IT IS EXCELLENT FOR
BRUNCH OR IN THE AFTERNOON AS A PICK-ME-UP WITH A CUP OF TEA OR COF-
FEE, OR YOU COULD FILL IT WITH PRESERVES AS IN THE CHOCOLATE LAYER
CAKE . IF YOU DO USE THE PRESERVES, SLICE THE CAKE CAREFULLY INTO TWO
LAYERS WITH A SERRATED KNIFE, AND THEN SPREAD THE PRESERVES OVER THE
BOTTOM LAYER. RASPBERRY IS ESPECIALLY FLAVORFUL.

Canola oil cooking spray
1 cup whole wheat pastry flour
1/2 cup brown sugar, firmly packed
10 egg whites, room temperature
1 teaspoon cream of tartar
Dash of salt
1/2 cup maple syrup
1/2 teaspoon maple or vanilla flavoring
1/4 cup almonds, toasted and finely chopped
Powdered sugar

Preheat the oven to 375°F. Spray a 10" tube pan with canola oil.
Dust with a little flour.
Sift the 1 cup flour and the brown sugar into a small bowl.
In a large metal bowl, beat the egg whites until soft peaks form.
Add the cream of tartar and salt, then slowly drizzle in the maple syrup,
beating to distribute the syrup evenly. Sift the flour mixture over the
egg mixture, 1/4 cup at a time, folding in gently. Fold in the flavoring
and almonds.
Spoon batter into the prepared tube pan. Bake for 35 minutes, or
until the top springs back when lightly touched. Invert in the pan and
cool.
Lift off the pan when cool and dust with powdered sugar.

Variations:

Honey Filbert: Follow the instructions above, substituting 1/3 cup honey for the maple syrup and 1/2 cup filberts for the almonds.

Lemon Poppy Seed: To the basic recipe add 1/4 cup poppy seeds, 1 teaspoon lemon flavoring in place of the vanilla, and 1 tablespoon grated lemon rind.

Calories per serving (basic recipe): 93. Percent of calories from fat 11%, protein 10%, carbohydrates 78%, 0 mg cholesterol.

☀ *Rice Pudding*

Serves 8

Served either warm or cold, this rice pudding is the basis for many creative variations. You can substitute 3 egg whites for the tofu, substitute dried apricots or prunes for the raisins, or omit the raisins and add 1/4 teaspoon grated fresh ginger and 1/4 cup toasted chopped almonds.

    Canola oil cooking spray
    1 cup brown rice
    1/2 cup raisins
    2 1/4 cups water
    1/2 cup blanched almonds (optional)
    3 cups low-fat or nonfat (skim) milk
    1 cup soft tofu
    1/4 cup maple syrup
    1 tablespoon vanilla
    3/4 teaspoon grated lemon rind
    1/4 teaspoon ground cinnamon
    1/4 teaspoon freshly grated nutmeg

Preheat the oven to 350°F.
Spray a 12" x 12" baking pan with canola oil.

Combine the rice with the raisins in 2 1/4 cups water in a medium saucepan. Bring to a boil, reduce the heat, cover, and simmer for 35 to 40 minutes, or until the rice is soft and the water absorbed.

In a food processor or blender, process the almonds with the milk and tofu for 1 minute. (If you prefer a creamy rice pudding, process until velvety smooth or omit the nuts) Pour into a bowl, add remaining ingredients, and stir well.

Pour the mixture into the prepared pan and bake for 50 minutes.

Calories per serving: 218. Percent of calories from fat 21%, protein 11%, carbohydrates 67%, 6 mg cholesterol.

☀ Noodle Kugel

Serves 8

THIS RECIPE DOUBLES EASILY AND IS GREAT FOR POTLUCKS OR BUFFET LUN-CHEONS. IT MAKES A GOOD DESSERT, BUT I ENJOY IT FOR A LUNCH ENTREE EVEN MORE.

8 ounces whole-wheat fettuccine noodles
1/2 cup low-fat or nonfat cottage cheese
1 egg plus 2 egg whites
1 cup plain nonfat yogurt
1/4 cup nonfat dry milk
3 tablespoons maple syrup,
   honey, or molasses
1 tablespoon lemon juice
1 teaspoon ground cinnamon
1/2 teaspoon nutmeg, freshly grated
1 teaspoon vanilla
1/3 cup raisins, soaked overnight
   in red wine and drained
1 large pear or apple, cored and chopped

Preheat the oven to 325°F. Spray a 12" baking pan or a 2-quart casserole dish with canola oil.

Cook the noodles according to package instructions. While they are boiling, whip the cottage cheese in a food processor until creamy. Place in a large pot and add all the remaining ingredients except the fruit. Blend well.

When the pasta is al dente, drain in a colander. Rinse under cold running water and drain thoroughly. Add to the cheese mixture and stir in the fruit. Blend well. Pour the kugel into the prepared pan and cover with foil.

Bake for 30 minutes. Remove the foil and bake for another 15 minutes, or until golden crust forms. Remove from the oven and cool.

While the kugel may be served warm, the flavors deepen when it is well chilled.

Calories per serving: 184. Percent of calories from fat 10%, protein 20%, carbohydrates 70%, 45 mg cholesterol.

✳ *Sweet Potato Pie*

Serves 8

BANANAS SWEETEN WHILE GINGER FLAVORS THIS UNUSUAL AND HIGHLY NUTRITIOUS PIE. IT'S WONDERFULLY RICH TASTING, AND WOULD DO WELL SERVED WITH SLIGHTLY TART FRESH GRAPES. A CUP OF CHOPPED NUTS IS GREAT STIRRED IN BEFORE BAKING — SAVE A FEW TO SPRINKLE ON TOP.

<u>Crust</u>
3/4 cup whole-wheat flour
1/4 cup walnuts, toasted and ground
1 tablespoon canola oil
1 tablespoon honey

<u>Filling</u>
2 pounds sweet potatoes, scrubbed
1 1/2 ripe bananas, peeled and sliced
2 green apples, peeled and chopped

2 tablespoons fresh ginger, minced
1/2 teaspoon cinnamon
1/2 cup apple juice
1/2 cup orange juice
1/4 cup lemon or lime juice
1 cup chopped nuts (optional)
Dash of salt
Canola oil cooking spray

Preheat the oven to 350°F.

Mix all the crust ingredients together with a pastry cutter or a fork until crumbly. Press the dough firmly and evenly into a deep-dish pie plate and chill for 20 minutes while you cook the sweet potatoes. Then prick the crust with a fork a half-dozen times. Bake for 20 minutes until golden brown.

Remove from the oven and cool, leaving the heat at 350°F.

Slice the potatoes into 1" rounds and place in a large saucepan with water to cover. Bring to a boil for 10 minutes, until soft. Drain and peel.

Meanwhile, spray a nonstick skillet with canola oil. Sauté the fruits together with the spices and salt over a low heat for 10 minutes, stirring frequently. In a food processor, puree the sweet potatoes, fruit juices, and half of the fruit. Pour into a bowl and stir in the remaining fruit and most of the nuts. Fill the pie crust evenly (and sprinkle with the remaining nuts.

Bake uncovered for 45 minutes.

Calories per serving (without nuts): 240. Percent of calories from fat 13%, protein 8%, carbohydrates 79%, 0 mg cholesterol.

✳ Tropical Dream Bars

Makes 2 dozen smaller bars
or 1 dozen larger bars

To SAVOR ALL OF THE WONDERFUL FLAVORS AND TEXTURES, THESE SWEET, SOFT BAR COOKIES SHOULD BE ENJOYED SLOWLY, WITH A TALL GLASS OF ICED TEA.

Canola oil cooking spray
1 egg plus 1 egg white
1/2 cup honey
1/2 cup evaporated skim milk
1 teaspoon vanilla
1 cup whole-wheat pastry flour
1 cup rolled oats
1/2 cup nonfat dry milk
1/2 cup wheat germ,
    lightly toasted
Dash of salt
    1/2 cup unsweetened shredded coconut
1/4 cup finely chopped dried papaya
1/4 cup finely chopped dried pineapple

Preheat the oven to 350°F. Spray an 8" x 8" baking pan with canola oil.

In a large bowl whip the egg, egg white, honey, evaporated skim milk, and vanilla to blend well.

In a medium-size bowl mix together the flour, oats, nonfat dry milk, wheat germ, and salt. Stir the dry ingredients into the wet until barely moistened. Add the coconut and dried fruit.

Spread the batter gently and evenly into the prepared pan. Do not pack it down. Bake for 7 minutes at the most. Remove from the oven and, when completely cool, cut into 12 or 24 bars.

Calories per 1 large bar or 2 small bars: 70. Percent of calories from fat 24%, protein 16%, carbohydrates 60%, 14 mg cholesterol.

Glossary of Foods

This dictionary will familiarize you with the foods that are used most often in the Anti-Aging Plan. In addition to describing the foods, we will refer you to recipes in which they are featured. If it is a food that you might not find in your local store, we have included mail order sources (see Appendix A). Most important, we will tell you what is so nutritionally remarkable about certain of these foods that makes them essential in the Anti-Aging Plan. We list foods with special nutrient values, herbs and spices that might be new to you, and foods from other countries that might enhance and facilitate nutrient-rich cooking.

The main goal of this dictionary and of this book is to offer the foods that are the most imortant for you to discover, use, understand, and above all, enjoy. We want foods such as cilantro, mung bean sprouts, couscous, nori, miso, wheat germ, brewer's yeast and the good old sweet potato or yam to become household words for you.

<u>Chinese Cabbage (Bok Choy)</u>:   This vegetable looks like a cross between celery and swiss chard. The stalks, which are generally sliced thinly and added to stir-fries, are sweet and crunchy. The leafy, dark-green tops cook more quickly and are delicious in soups. Calorie for calorie they are higher in calcium than any other vegetable.

<u>Broccoli</u>: Broccoli is a cruciferous superfood vegetable known for its antioxidant benefits in the form of vitamin C and beta-carotene as well as its colon and rectal cancer-fighting agents. One medium stalk contains only 56 calories,along with 6 grams of protein, .5 grams of fat, 330 percent of your daily requirements for vitamin C, 90 percent for vitamin A, 500 percent for vitamin K, 11 percent for iron, and 15 percent for calcium.

<u>Brewer's Yeast</u>: Brewer's yeast is a super-charger food that appears in many recipes. Please refer to Page 97 for a complete explanation of brewer's yeast.

<u>Capers</u>: Capers are small green pickled buds of a flowering Mediterranean bush. They are used to flavor fish and dressings.

Cardamom: This is an invaluable spice of the ginger family used in Indian, Indonesian, and Middle Eastern cooking. It is sweetly aromatic and, in minute quantities, will flavor custards, apples, and peaches as well as in the recipes included here.

Chard, Swiss or Red: In the leafy green family of superfoods, 4 ounces of chard, 28 calories, will supply you with 61 percent of your RDAs for vitamin C, 150 percent for vitamin A, 37 percent for manganese, 34 percent for potassium, and 20 percent for iron. Swiss chard can be pureed into a sauce, and use it instead of spinach in Greens Soup. Also, try Sherried Swiss Chard.

Cilantro: These green, aromatic leave of the coriander plant lie side by side with parsley in your supermarket. Used abundantly in Mexican and Asian cooking, it perks up salads, salsas, and makes an excellent garnish for fish.

Coriander, Ground: Mild and sweet, yet slightly pungent, this spice is used extensively in Asian cooking.

Cottage Cheese, Low- or Nonfat: Common cottage cheese is a versatile superfood on our list. High in protein (14 g) and low in fat (3 g) 1/2 cup of low-fat cottage cheese contains 110 calories and can easily be whipped into an excellent topping for baked potatoes or used as a salad dressing (see Guacamole). One-half cup supplies 24 percent of your daily needs for vitamin B12 (a difficult requirement when minimizing red meat on your dinner table), 13 percent for selenium, and 60 percent for vitamin K. For a high-protein lunch, try our Cheese Salad.

Garlic: Used throughout the world, garlic has a lore that makes it mythic. Fresh garlic is essential. Choose heads that are plump and firm, not grey, soggy, or soft. Store in a cool, dry place with adequate ventilation. Refrigeration is not recommended. To peel garlic, press each clove against the cutting board with the side of a broad knife. Once slightly squashed, the skin will slip off easily.

Garlic flavors food differently, depending on how it is cooked. Raw garlic used in pesto, for example, is quite strong and becomes more so with time. When sautéing garlic, take care not to burn it. Garlic chips roasted in the oven make good toppings on salads and baked potatoes. Whole cloves added to stews and roasts lend a milder flavor.

Ginger: Fresh ginger is a spicy, hot, and pungent knobby rhizome. Its uses are many. In marinades, sauces, stir-fries, and Asian cooking, its zippy flavor is not as hot as chili. Peel away the outer skin and mince or grate.

Kale: Of the calcium- and iron-rich dark leafy green family, 4 ounces of kale contains a mere 43 calories. It is heavily armed with your daily nutritional needs for four potent antioxidants: vitamin C (240%), vitamin A (205%), vitamin E (61%), and selenium (41%). With an additonal 19% of your RDAs for iron and 9 % for calcium, kale is also high in potassium, manganese, and magnesium. To make it a regular visitor at your table, try using it in place of the spinach in our Spinach and Roasted Garlic (see recipe page 270), or sample Shiitake Mushrooms and Greens (see recipe page 269)

Kombu: Kombu seaweed is a super-charger food we frequently add to our stews and greens. Please refer to page 95 for a complete nutritional description and preparation instructions.

Milk, Nonfat: In our computer-generated meal plans, calcium was one of the most difficult requirements to fill. One cup of skim milk, only 85 calories, features 25 percent of your RDA for calcium, 31 percent of vitamin B12, and 22 percent of riboflavin, selenium, phosphorus, potassium, and vitamin D. For an action-packed shake, try 1 cup of skim milk, 1 banana, 1/4 tsp vanilla-flavoring and 1 tablespoon of wheat germ.

Milk, Nonfat Dry: The instant nonfat dry milk found in your supermarket is another super-charger food. You will find an explanation of its many valuable properties in Chapter 9.

Mirin: Mirin is a sweet sake used in many marinades, soups, and stir-fries. Pale dry sherry may be substituted , or regular sake may be slightly sweetened. Mirin's alcohol content evaporates in the cooking process.

Mustard seeds, black: Used primarily in Indian curries and soups, they are usually roasted to release their nutty flavor before being added to a recipe. In texture, they are similiar to poppy seeds.

Miso: Miso is a fermented soybean paste used as a flavoring in soups and as a dressing or marinade. Its sodium content is high, and thus should be avoided by those monitoring salt intake. It can be found in the Asian section of your market.

Nori: Also known as laver or sea lettuce, nori is the paper-thin dark green sheet of seaweed wrapped around your sushi roll. It is a super-charger food. Please refer to page 96 for tips on its nutrient value and preparation.

Okra: Sometimes called gumbo, and a main ingredient in Creole cooking, okra is a member of the hibiscus family. The pods are harvested when quite young, while still small and sweet. If not available fresh, frozen okra is generally available. Prized as a thickener in stews and soups, do not let its slipperiness daunt you. If cooking the vegetable solo, avoid piercing the pods, and cook them until just tender. This will minimize viscosity. They can be steamed, sauteed, and added to stews and casseroles.

Paprika: Is made from dried, ground, sweet red peppers. Hot paprika can be used in place of cayenne.

Saffron: Used classically in Spanish paella, saffron is an aromatic spice providing a bright yellow color and delicate, pungent flavor. Saffron threads, the world's most expensive spice, are the hand-picked stamens of the crocus flowers. It takes more than 70,000 flowers to produce 1 pound of saffron, but a little goes a long way in any recipe.

Shiitake mushrooms: You will frequently find these meaty, elegant and nutritious mushrooms in my refrigerator. They are a super-charger food well worth discovering. Please refer to Chapter 9 for complete directions on how to find them, on their preparation, and for their nutrient values.

Soba Noodles: These are thin spaghetti like noodles made from buckwheat and sometimes wheat flour. The amount of buckwheat flour
varies. Try to use 100% buckwheat. Their uniquely nutty flavor is a
welcome alternative to spaghetti.

Soybeans: These beans are a potent super-charger food now available
in many commercialy prepared forms. For more information, please
refer to Chapter 9.

Spinach: Stock your refridgerator regularly with spinach. In 1/4 lb you
will find 40 calories and four potent anti-oxidents: 100% of your RDA's
for vitamin C, 186% for vitamin A, 41% for selenium, and 21% for
vitamin E.   1/4 lb of spinach will also fill your daily needs for: iron,
19%; vitamin K, 146%, and calcium, 9%.

Sweet Potato: On a nutrional scoreboard compiled by the Center for
Science in the Public Interest (Nutrition Action Health Letter, December
1991) comparing values for eight nutrients to access the healthiest
vegetables, seet potatoes topped the list._There are 100 calories in one
half of one sweet potato. With 100 percent of your requirements for
vitamen A, 40 percent for vitamen E, and 30 percent for vitamin C, the
sweet potato is a free radical fighter.

Tahini: Tahini is a paste similiar to peanut butter, made from hulled and
toasted sesame seeds. Oil content in seeds is lower than in nut butters,
but is still relatively high. Hence, tahini should be used sparingly. It
can be thinned out with yogurt, tofu, or miso depending on the recipe.
Nutritionally, sesame seeds are loaded with vitamin E.

Thickeners (Arrowroot and Cornstarch): These two are practically
interchangeable and are excellent alternatives to a butter-based flour
roux. Both should be mixed with a small amount of cold broth or water
before being added to your recipe. Arrowroot's translucency is better
suited for vegetable-based sauces while the cornstarch is slighty milky.
Cornstarch freezes better, however, and will not separate upon reheating.

<u>Tofu</u>: Tofu is yet another super-charger food. Please refer to page 98 for a description of the wonderful features in tofu.

<u>Turnip Greens</u>: Turnip greens are the most nutrient packed of all the green leafy vegetables. The numbers speak for themselves, RDA % in 4 ounces: Vitamin C - 200 percent, Vitamin A - 175 percent, Manganese - 65 percent, Vitamin E - 25 percent, Vitamin B2 - 25 per-cent, Calcium - 25 percent, and Iron - 11 percent. Substitute them for the cooked spinach in your favorite recipe.

Vinegars:
<u>Balsamic</u>: This is our favorite, and it has recently become increasingly popular. Although slightly more expensive, its distinctive flavor height-ens salads and marinades alike. Add a 1/4 teaspoon and a sprinkle of sesame seeds to steamed greens for a real treat.   <u>Rice</u>: Lighter and more delicate than the others, rice vinegar is ideal on pasta salads, and in many salad dressings.   <u>Fruit Vinegars</u>: Raspberry, peach, and cur-rants, to name but a few, are relatively new to the home chef. Include at least one flavor on your shelf for salads requesting a tart dressing (say, with shrimp salads, or with feta cheese).

<u>Wheat germ</u>: This is such a special super-charged food that it deserves a special place in your diet. Please refer to page 99 for many sugges-tions on how and why you should add this food daily to your diet.

<u>Yogurt, Lowfat or Nonfat</u>:   One cup of nonfat yogurt, 100 calories, boasts 37 percent of your daily needs for calcium. Yogurt is perhaps the richest source for calcium, calorie for calorie. That same 1 cup bears 49 percent of your RDAs for vitamin B12 and 30 percent for riboflavin. The protein/fat ratio is 4 to 1; there are no empty calories in nonfat yogurt! We have used it in 20 percent of our recipes,either as a main ingredient or as a nutrient enrichening addition.

Appendix A
Special Food Sources

<u>Walnut Acres</u>: You will find almost everything you need from this company. Penn Creek, PA 17863. (800) 433-3998.

<u>International Selection</u>: This is a good source for seaweed and shiitake mushrooms. P.O. Box 3163, Fort Lee, NJ 07024 (800) 253-1672

<u>Williams Sonoma</u>: For vinegars and gourmet selections.
P.O. Box 7456, San Francisco, CA 94120.

Appendix B
Cooking With a Personal Computer

Cooking can be both a creative and a relaxing art, with endless variations. And with recent trends toward a healthier diet, you are probably familiar with low-fat cuisine. But what makes the Anti-Aging Plan's health program unique are the fortifying benefits of a nutrient-rich diet. The only way truly to design such a program is with a computer.

For the last two years the computer has taught the authors of this book more about what we put into our bodies than we could have imagined. It has shaped the way we think about food today. Our meals have become as nourishing to our bodies as they are satisfying to our palates. These recipes were put together between the hard disk on our computers and the skillet. Truly a diet for the twenty-first century!

Notice that most of the nutrient-rich Megameal recipes in Chapter 10 have a larger number of ingredients than the standard versions of these same recipes that you will find in cookbooks. Let us explain how these recipes came about.

We began by typing a standard recipe into the computer program that became Dr. Walford's Interactive Diet Planner. To simplify our work, we began by entering a recipe to feed one person.

With a few key strokes, the computer gave us a calorie, fat, and protein count; the percentage of calories from fat, protein, and carbohydrate; and the cholesterol level. It also told us the percentage of the Recommended Daily Allowance for amino acids, vitamins, and minerals in those foods. We were really surprised to see how nutritionally unbalanced most recipes actually are — even the "healthy" ones, those that feature reduced fat or a low calorie count. Unless a wide variety of foods was included, the vitamin and mineral count usually suffered.

Seeing that the meal we were planning lacked, for instance, selenium, vitamin E, vitamin B6, zinc, and calcium, we would proceed to the Search Routine. It was here that we learned the most about nutrition. We could, for instance, ask the computer to itemize only vegetables that are high in selenium, vitamin E, and vitamin B6. We learned that while sweet potatoes and kale are good sources for vitamin E, vegetables are really not carriers for selenium or vitamin B6. Running the search program again, we learned that seaweeds are a great source for vitamin B6, while whole wheat, sunflower seeds, wheat germ, and many fishes are high in selenium

We hunted the computer database for nutrient-rich superfoods, even if they seemed foreign, or unusual. Seaweeds, okay. We experimented with nori torn up in salads, and kombu soaked and added to stews, casseroles, or just about anything cooked. We learned what our tastebuds liked. We grew to savor the deep green spots of salty nori in our salads; while a winter broth made from kombu (used as a staple in Asia the way we use chicken broth) would perk us right up.

Juggling between energy intensity (calories) and nutrient density, we looked not only at the amount of selenium per serving portion, but also at calorie counts. One tablespoon of wheat germ contains only 33 calories and 13 percent of the Recommended Daily Allowances for selenium, while 1 tablespoon of sunflower seeds also contains 13 percent of your requirements for selenium but twice as many calories! So wheat germ contains, on a calorie to nutrient ratio, twice as much selenium as sunflower seeds. We would go through the same process for zinc, calcium, or whatever nutrient we lacked.

As we became more familiar with them, we learned the supercharger foods that we could squeeze into almost any recipe to hike it's nutrient density. As you will notice from the recipes, we added wheat germ, seaweeds, and brewer's yeast whenever possible. While not changing the flavor of these dishes, these three foods greatly enhance the nutritional profile of each recipe.

Simply, the computer showed us food combinations that met our nutritional specifications. From there, we could reshape a casserole into a quiche by reducing the liquid and adding a nutritious crust. Or we could modify it into a rolled burrito or baked crepes simply by changing the seasonings and the method of preparation. The actual ingredients would remain the same.

The restrictions that we placed on a recipe or that you place on your diet will determine which nutrient values will be hardest to fill. For instance, when developing vegetarian combinations, we were low in B vitamins, and in iron. If we further omitted dairy, calcium and vitamin D were lacking! My vegetarian friends supplement their recipes with seaweeds, which can more than adequately fill the Recommended Daily Allowances for some B vitamins. Two grams of nori (one 4" x 6" sheet, easily a single serving when mixed with a salad or casserole) contains 27 percent of your vitamin D (tough on a dairy-free diet), and only 4 calories! Seaweeds are, however, a poor substitute for dairy. Two grams will give you only 2 percent of your calcium requirements. Leafy greens, while virtually empty of B vitamins, are high in calcium. Four ounces of turnip greens (about 1 cup steamed) contain only 28 calories but will give you 24 percent of your daily requirements for calcium, 11 percent for iron, a whopping 232 percent for vitamin C, and 152 percent for vitamin A. So we would add nori to our recipe, and perhaps make a sauce with the greens or serve them creamed with yogurt as a side dish. Our daily needs for B vitamins, calcium, iron, vitamins C, K, and A have practically been fulfilled while adding only 28 calories!

As you can see, this process is mathematical, and would be impossible to do accurately without a computer.

Armed with facts, we began to look at our own "healthy" diet. We had already begun reducing our fat and caloric intake, but had very little understanding of how to develop a nutrient-rich plan. Now, in addition to incorporating wheat germ, brewer's yeast, and seaweeds into our recipes, we regularly include such foods as bananas, broccoli, red peppers, greens of all types, tofu, wild rice, sardines, oysters, salmon, oat bran, nonfat (skim) milk, nonfat yogurt, calves liver, and grains of all kinds.

The Megemeals in Chapter 10 were designed using this computer program. They emphasize taste and familiarity with the health benefits of carefully selected food combinations.

Dr. Walford's Interactive Diet Planner is available for purchase to help you design your own Megameals. The program features over 1,200 foods including name-brand, processed, and fast foods. Fats are broken down into polyunsaturated, monounsaturated, and saturated. You can even personalize your daily vitamin and mineral allowances to some figure other than those commonly recommended.

The program comes in a Windows and a DOS version with a graphic, color display and an expandable database. Installation is simple, and an instruction manual with a quick reference quide walks you through the various features of the software. No special knowledge is needed to use this program. A Macintosh program is forthcoming.

The Interactive Diet Planner is available through the Longbrook Company, 1015 Gayley Avenue, Suite 1215, Los Angeles, CA. 90024 (310) 392-8208.

Appendix C
Sample Menus

An asterisk * means that the recipe appears in this book.

First Day
Breakfast
1 Baked Apple* (330 calories)
1/4 cup low-fat cottage cheese (45)
coffee or tea

Lunch
1 Super Burrito* (517)
1 glass skim milk blended with 1 banana (banana shake) (140)

Dinner
3 oz. broiled salmon, halibut or swordfish (220)
1/2 baked potato (96) topped with 1/3 cup Creamy Garlic Sauce* (52)

3/4 cup cooked green peas and carrots (90)

Snack
1 slice Spiced Honey Cake* (118)

Second Day
Breakfast
3/4 cup fat-free dry cereal with 1 cup lowfat milk (185)
1 banana (100)
coffee or tea

Lunch
2 slices whole wheat bread with 3 oz. turkey breast, tomato, lettuce,
mustard and 1 sliced egg white (260)
fruit shake with 1 cup nonfat yogurt and 1/2 cup berries (140)

Dinner
1 serving Watercress soup* (31)
1 serving Chow Mein* (605)

Snack
1 apple (85)
1 cup hot or whipped skim milk with nutmeg, saffron, and 1/2 tsp
honey (100)

Third Day
Breakfast
1 slice toasted fat-free whole wheat bread (60)
1 poached egg (80)
1 glass orange juice (112)
coffee or tea

Lunch
1 Stuffed Green Pepper* (384)
1/2 cup nonfat yogurt with 1 tsp fruit-only jam or honey (60)

Dinner
2 oz. lean pork chop, broiled with 1/2 cup unsweetened apple sauce (130)
1/2 cup mashed potato with 1 tblsp lowfat cottage cheese (80)
1 stalk steamed broccoli (60)

Snack
1 tropical dream bar* (70)
a glass skim milk (85)

Fourth Day

Breakfast
2 Buckwheat Pancakes* (120)
1/2 cup sliced fresh fruit or 2 tblsp raisins (50)
1 glass skim milk (85)
coffee or tea

Lunch
1 pita pocket sandwich with 1/3 cup Hummus*, tomato, lettuce (290)
1 cup tomato juice (50)
1/2 cup grapes or 2 tblsp raisins (50)

Dinner
1 slice Pâté with Velvet Sauce* (492)
Tossed green salad with tomato, cucumber, scallions, 1 tsp. Poppy Seed Dressing* (100)

Snack
1 cup frozen berries (75)
1/4 cup nonfat yogurt with 1/2 tsp honey (50)
2 graham crackers (60)

Fifth Day

Breakfast
1/3 cup rolled oats with 1/2 tsp yeast (108)
1/2 cup buttermilk, 1/2 cup skim milk and 1/2 banana blended

together (130)
2 prunes or 2 dried apricots (50)

Lunch
3 oz. roasted chicken (155)
2 slices fat-free whole wheat bread with tomato, lettuce, onion, mustard (140)
1 glass skim milk (85)
1 Tropical Dreambar* (70)

Dinner
Mussels Florentine* (419)
1 stalk steamed broccoli with 1/2 roasted or steamed red pepper
(73)

Snack
1 slice Sweet Potato Pie* (240)
1 glass skim milk (85)

Sixth Day

Breakfast
Scrambled Eggs* (mostly egg whites; see recipe; 117)
1 corn muffin (140)
a glass skim milk (85)

Lunch
1 slice toasted raisin bread (70)
with 1 tblsp peanut butter and 1/4 thinly sliced apple (95)
1 cup nonfat yogurt mixed with 1/2 cup berries (150)

Dinner
Classic Paella* (540)
Mixed salad of carrots, radishes, spinach, cucumbers and cabbage
with 1/4 clove pressed garlic and 2 tblsp nonfat yogurt (50)
1 glass nonfat milk (85)

Snack

1 apple with 1/4 cup lowfat cottage cheese topped with 1 tblsp
toasted wheat germ (110)

Seventh Day

Breakfast
French Toast with 1/2 cup pureed fruit (256)
1 glass nonfat milk (85)

Lunch
1 serving Vegetarian Quiche* (447)
1 apple (85)

Dinner
3 oz. broiled chicken breast (155)
1 cup whole wheat pasta with Pesto* sauce (200)
Steamed 1/2 carrot and 1/2 stalk broccoli (65)

Snack
1 slice Chocolate Layer Cake* (157)
1 glass nonfat milk (85)

Eighth Day

Breakfast
1 soft-boiled egg (90)
1 slice whole wheat bread with a thin slice of low-fat mozzarella (93)
1 glass skim milk (85)

Lunch
1 serving Cheese Salad* with 1 whole wheat roll (230)
1 orange (90)

Dinner
1 Tostada* (500)
1 glass skim milk (85)
1 cup grapes (100)

Snack
1/2 Sliced peach served with 1/2 cup yogurt (78)

Appendix D
Bibliography

Other Books By Roy L. Walford

The Retardation of Aging And Desease By Dietary Restriction with Richard Weindruch, Ph.D.   Springfield, Illinois; Charles C. Thomas, 1988.

The 120-Year Diet: How to Double Your Vital Years. New York: Simon & Shuster, 1986; New York: Pocket Books, 1988 (paperback)

Maximum Lifespan. New York: W. W. Norton, 1983; New York: Avon Books, 1983 (paperback)

Other Reading
Carper, Jean.   **Food Your Miracle Medicine.**   New York: Harper Collins, 1993.

Carper, Jean. **The Food Pharmacy.** New York: Bantam, 1989.

Hoshijo, Kathy. **Kathy Cooks.** New York: Simon & Shuster, 1989.

Murray, Michael M.D. **The Healing Power Of Foods.**   Rochlin, Ca.: Prima Publishing, 1993.

Ornish, Dean, M.D. **Dr. Dean Ornish's Program for Revising Heart Disease.** New York: Ballantine, 1992

Penn State University.   **Heart Healthy Shopping Guide** is a pocket guide on low-fat/low-cholesterol foods. Contact: Penn State Nutrition Center, 417 East Calder Way, Pennsylvania State University, University

Park, PA 16801-5663.

Light & Healthy Cook Book. The Best Of Sunset. Menlo Park, Ca.: Sunset Publishing Corporation, 1990.

For Nutrient Tables
Carper, Jean. **Total Nutrition Guide**. New York: Bantam Books, 1987.

Lavon, Dunn. **Nutrition Almanac**. New York: McGraw-Hill, 1990.

National Research Council. **Recommended Dietary Allowances, 10th Ed.** Washington D.C.: National Academy Press, 1989.

Newsletters
Center For Science In The Public Interest. *Nutrition Action Health Letter*. 1875 Connecticut Ave., N.W. Suite 300, Washington D.C. 20009-5728.

Tufts University Diet and Nutrition Letter. 53 Park Place, N.Y., NY10007

Cooking Light, The Magazine Of Food And Fitness, published bimonthly by Southern Living. (800) 336-0125

Index